GUT INSTINCT

WHAT YOUR STOMACH IS TRYING TO TELL YOU

GUT INSTINCT

WHAT YOUR STOMACH IS TRYING TO TELL YOU

7 EASY STEPS TO HEALTH AND HEALING

Pierre Pallardy

RODALE

This edition first published in the UK in 2006 by
Rodale International Ltd
7–10 Chandos Street
London W1G 9AD
www.rodalebooks.co.uk

This book was originally published in French as *Et si ça venait du ventre?* by Editions
Robert Laffont, SA, Paris, 2002

English translation by Translate-A-Book, Oxford, England

Book design by Paul Ashby

Cover photograph by Corbis

Printed and bound in the UK by CPI Bath using acid-free paper from sustainable
sources.

1 3 5 7 9 8 6 4 2

A CIP record for this book is available from the British Library

ISBN-10: 1-4050-9977-1
ISBN-13: 978-1-4050-9977-6

This paperback edition distributed to the book trade by Pan Macmillan Ltd

Notice
This book is intended as a reference volume only, not as a medical manual. The
information given here is designed to help you make informed decisions about your
health. It is not intended as a substitute for any treatment that you may have been
prescribed by your doctor. If you suspect that you have a medical problem, we urge
you to seek competent medical help.

Mention of specific companies, organisations or authorities in this book does not
imply endorsement by the publisher, nor does mention of specific companies,
organisations or authorities in the book imply that they endorse the book.

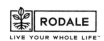

LIVE YOUR WHOLE LIFE™

We inspire and enable people to improve their lives and the world around them

This book is dedicated to therapists, osteopaths, nurses, midwives and medical practitioners everywhere – in short, to all those who use a hands-on approach to alleviate their patients' suffering and guide them back along the often difficult path to health and well-being.

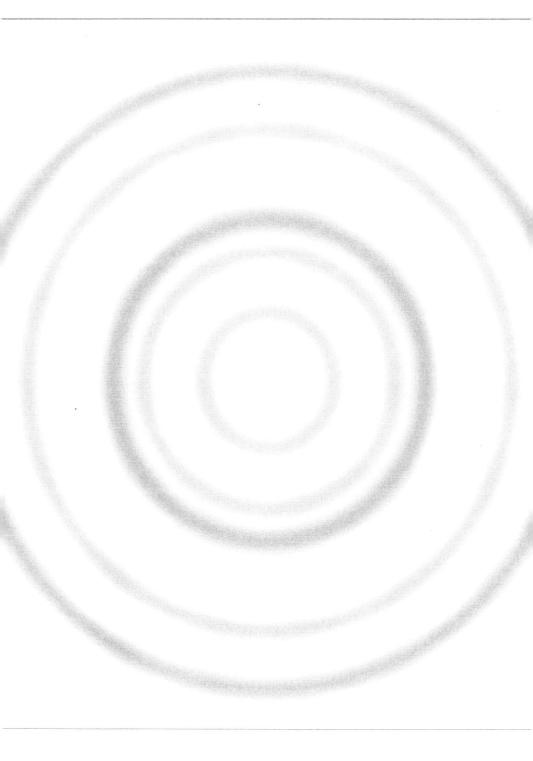

CONTENTS

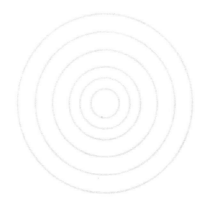

INTRODUCTION

OVER MANY YEARS, MY VOCATION as a therapist has brought me into contact with countless patients plagued by all manner of physical and psychological complaints, which have caused them great suffering. In some cases, they felt their lives were almost not worth living. Each one has sought a solution to their problems, determined to find a means of achieving that special feeling of harmony and happiness that comes from the health and well-being that should be our birthright.

In almost every single instance, there was little need to delve into their medical history: I could read it in their eyes. These were patients in distress, patients who had consulted one specialist after another, patients who had followed strict diets and experimented with every treatment under the sun, eagerly espousing each and every 'miracle' cure that came on the market and dutifully swallowing everything from anti-depressants to mega-vitamins. Typically, they tried whatever was on offer in a despairing bid to find some means of putting an end to their discomfort and suffering.

The stresses and strains of modern life are all around us. We are plagued by the speed of events, which offer little scope for relaxation. We eat too quickly, whenever or wherever we can, consuming food without regard to its nutritional value. We eat too much sugar. We eat too many fatty foods. At times, in an attempt to remedy an unhealthy lifestyle, we indulge in sporadic exercise, turning to sports that are often too extreme or, at best, poorly adapted to our physical needs. Nothing seems to work. We remain exhausted. We sleep badly. We are out of condition, overweight, tortured by back pain. We accumulate allergies, we suffer from rheumatism and arthritis, we develop sexual problems, such as impotence or loss of libido. All too often, I can see the first signs of premature ageing on a patient's face. And, in the vast majority of instances, I detect the spiral of stress that leads inexorably down towards depression.

This makes me angry. As a practising osteopath, dietician and physiotherapist with 35 years of clinical experience, I know that almost all these physical and mental ailments could have been avoided in the first instance and, once established, can still be successfully treated and cured. The sole pre-condition is a willingness to eliminate certain bad habits, to eat sensibly and to change the way you breathe; my simple set of behavioural rules will also change the way in which you perceive yourself. It is simply a question of understanding that complaints such as those outlined above are almost exclusively abdomen-related. They have their origins in the abdomen and it is there that a cure must be sought.

To put it bluntly, we must learn to trust our gut instincts.

The Abdomen as Epicentre

On the face of it, asserting that everything relates back to the abdomen may not appear particularly logical or even defensible. Since my early days as a practising therapist, however, I have believed that treating the abdomen is an essential part of the therapeutic process. I would even go so far as to say that the abdomen is the epicentre of life. Throughout my career, my first reflex has always been to seek a remedy by adopting a hands-on approach to the abdomen, regardless of the patient's initial complaint.

In my very first book, *La grande forme* ('Top Form', published in 1979), I stressed the importance of maintaining the abdomen in the best possible condition and getting plenty of oxygen to the area. In 1981, in *En pleine santé* ('Total Health'), I traced the close links between recurrent complaints and abdominal dysfunction. Then, in *Manger pour guérir* ('Eating for Health', published in 1985), I set out a basic method for achieving a sense of well-being. I quote *Manger pour guérir*:

For over twenty years, patients have been coming to me on a daily basis complaining of back and neck pain, of aching joints, of sleeping disorders, of a general feeling of lassitude and exhaustion. Some have described excruciatingly painful migraines, others have protested that their nerves were frayed to the point where they were unable to carry on. Without fail, when I examined their back, neck and limbs, I immediately detected signs of knots and tension. But when I palpated their abdomen, I also discovered that the area was hard, bloated, under stress. Typically, severe pain manifested itself at certain points on the plexus – that complex network of minute and closely interwoven and interconnecting fibres and tubes – and along certain meridians, the pathways in the body along which energy flows. I would treat the patient by gently massaging the abdomen, progressively releasing the knots of tension. As I proceeded, I could feel the patient gradually relax as his or her condition improved.

In *Maigrir sans regrossir* ('Slimming for Good', 2000), I took issue with formal dieting, advocating in its place the principle of 'oxygenation' based on a 'breathe-to-relax' method that directly affects the digestive system. I showed that my method could lead not only to sustained weight loss but also to a reduction in physical

...most back problems, including recurrent sciatica, chronic lumbar disorders, neuralgia and rheumatism, could be alleviated by developing a healthy abdominal structure...

malfunction as a whole and, notably, it could act as an antidote to insomnia, fatigue, skin complaints, depression and allergies.

Not least, in *Plus jamais mal au dos* ('An End to Back Pain', 2001) – a study that proved an eye-opener in many circles, not least among top-level athletes – I argued that most back problems, including recurrent sciatica, chronic lumbar disorders, neuralgia and rheumatism, could be alleviated by developing a healthy abdominal structure by using my breathe-to-relax therapy and paying attention to nutrition. Over time, personal experience confirmed my professional convictions.

In my view, the abdomen is much more than a collection of pipes and tubes that serve the process of digestion and elimination of waste material and toxins. Instead, I have long asserted that the abdomen is actually a 'second brain', which plays a crucial role in sustaining health and well-being.

I recall the scepticism with which some of my patients – and, indeed, many of my colleagues – greeted this notion, but I clung stubbornly to the view that there was little to be gained by treating a complaint at the purely local level. Instead, priority should be given to the abdomen. In ancient times, I would point out, the stomach was widely held to be the 'seat of the soul', and the abdomen was the prime focus of Oriental medicine. Chinese practitioners were in the habit of examining a patient's abdomen by monitoring the pulse or listening to the heartbeat. I would refer doubting Thomases to the modest but growing body of medical literature identifying the abdomen as an organ that produces immune cells, similar in quantity to those produced by spinal cord marrow.

No matter what I said, however, my ideas were initially greeted with polite scepticism (at best). I achieved some spectacular results, but even those failed to convince the doubters. One case involved a leading practitioner from a teaching hospital who was suffering from a cervico-brachial neuritis (nerve inflammation), which manifested itself in the form of shoulder pain that stubbornly refused to respond to treatment. He had consulted several of his colleagues and submitted to various therapies, including anti-inflammatory drugs, poultices, massage and manipulation – all to no avail. On examining him, I discovered his stomach was in a pitiful state. I treated him to several sessions of abdominal massage, outlawed his daily coffee intake (six or seven cups), insisted that he take regular meals (to be ingested slowly) and instructed him to follow my breathe-to-relax method. Without directly treating his painful shoulder, I succeeded in significantly improving his overall condition. He continues to be grateful to this day.

No matter: I was still preaching to the unconverted.

Then, out of the blue in the early years of the 21st century, articles began to appear in venerable medical journals, notably in the United States. Exhaustive research had come up with one or two startling conclusions, among them the following:

- The abdomen is both structurally and neuro-chemically a 'second brain' connected directly to and complementing the upper brain.
- The intestine produces between 70 and 85 per cent of the body's immune cells, affording protection against serious illness.
- The abdomen generates interstitial cells (those that go in the gaps between bones and tissues), which play a vital role in the proper functioning of muscles and articulation of joints.
- The abdomen boasts a complex and hitherto unsuspected network of molecular neuro-transmitters ('nerve-messengers', if you will) and modulators identical to those generated by the upper brain. To date, these include some 30 substances, such as serotonin, melatonin, acetylcholine and epinephrin.

Next, Michael D. Gershon, a professor at New York's Columbia University and a specialist in anatomy and cellular biology, published a study based on 30 years of research. The impact of his book *The Second Brain*[1] was nothing short of sensational.

Gershon argued that the two brains, the 'upper' brain and the 'abdominal' brain, must work in tandem, or there will be 'chaos' in the abdomen and 'misery' in the head. In essence, Gershon's research demonstrated the existence of a reciprocal chemistry operating between these two brains via the vagus nerve, which supplies the upper digestive tract and the organs of the chest cavity and abdomen. In consequence, the abdomen has the ability to register tastes. Since then, a team from Boston University[2] has identified in the stomach and the intestinal ligament a series of receptors capable of detecting 'a bitter taste'.

The Second Brain adduced clear scientific evidence of what I had concluded solely on the basis of intuition, namely that treating the abdomen and reinstating any functions which had been altered or modified by disorders such as gastritis, colitis, constipation or diarrhoea will exert a positive, relaxing and curative effect on the patient. It also boosts the body's natural defence system and protects it against infection. To be honest, even my own boldest conjectures do not go as far as those of Professor Gershon, who – to cite an example given in *The Second Brain* – asserts that the type of blood platelets that develop when a patient has Alzheimer's or Parkinson's diseases comes from both the upper brain and the intestines.

Reading Gershon's book helped me understand why my method of treating the abdomen also improves the functioning of the cardiovascular system and is effective in treating diabetes, regulating blood flow, reducing cholesterol and dissipating muscular and rheumatoid pain. These beneficial effects also extend to mental disorders such as anxiety and depression, which are linked to serotonin, a molecule secreted by both brains.

Immunity and the Abdomen

When manipulating a patient's abdomen, I have frequently observed that the procedure has something in common with psychiatry or psychoanalysis, bringing to the surface deep-rooted emotions and traumas that may have been repressed since early childhood. At times, I have been astonished to find patients suddenly confiding in me. It seems that, in the process of working on a painful area, I have somehow tapped into the previously hidden well-springs of the subconscious, triggering an unexpected recollection. Working the abdomen has touched a sensitive nerve that, in turn, has resulted in an involuntary fit of trembling, spasms and tears. It is as if lost memories come to the surface, prompting a flood of confidences.

At this stage, reactions such as these have long since ceased to surprise me, not least because I am alert to the role of neurotransmitters originating in the abdomen and to the vital links that exist between the two brains. This process of 'inter-connectivity' is one I suspect the founding fathers of psychoanalysis must have sensed. I have read that both Freud and Jung were in the habit of placing their hands on a patient's head and abdomen during consultations. It has also been recorded that, in his early days, Freud used to massage a subject's abdomen during treatment. I have often contrived to put my patients at their ease and to dispel or partially alleviate their fears. It is now eminently clear to me that my ministrations have proved successful when a sense of harmony and equilibrium between the two brains has been established. Alleviation of nervous disorders is often followed by a quite spectacular physical improvement, notably reduced incidence of insomnia, depression or sexual difficulties.

A malfunctioning abdomen is responsible for many disorders, such as back pain, fatigue, insomnia or skin complaints, which we would not automatically associate with that organ (see Part III). The principal purpose of this book is to place at the reader's disposal a method, developed painstakingly over the years, of dealing with respiratory and alimentary aspects of the abdomen in order to develop and sustain its health and to promote harmony between this second brain and the upper brain. This method will help the reader address numerous common ailments, which are listed alphabetically in Part III. I would add only that I have somehow always known that the method 'works' in practice; now, however, I understand why it works. And, as a therapist, I may perhaps be forgiven for taking some pride in the fact that my instincts in this respect preceded scientific proof by close on three decades.

The principal purpose of this book is to place at the reader's disposal a method... of dealing with respiratory and alimentary aspects of the abdomen to develop and sustain its health...

The abdomen has come of age and emerged from the twilight zone it once occupied in 'polite' society. Fashions change: skirts and trousers are cut lower on the waist, stomachs are exposed and navels are pierced with increasing frequency. 'Belly-dancing' is in vogue, and magazines have begun featuring the rounded silhouettes of pregnant women in their pages. This shift in perceptions and attitudes is mirrored in patient behaviour. When I first started in practice – well before I graduated as an osteopath – I was conscious that patients reacted with instinctive reticence as soon as my hands touched their abdomen. This was particularly true of female patients. It was if I was somehow trespassing on their intimacy, venturing across a frontier into a 'no-go' area. Today, that is no longer the case; male and female patients automatically accept and respond positively to the touch of the therapist's hand, even if there is an initial, not inconsiderable level of pain when I first start kneading the plexus and exploring the disposition of the intestine, colon, liver or gall bladder.

The Potential of the Second Brain

The impact of the method I describe in this book is diverse and far-reaching. I believe that treating the abdomen with the respect it deserves goes a long way towards protecting it against the risks presented by our consumer society. By improving both the quantity and quality of our body's immune cell make-up, there is a strong chance that we can decrease the risks of developing cancerous tumours.

It is an established fact in more affluent societies, where quality of life expectations are increasingly higher, that one in two of us is liable to experience some form of cancer. My method of conditioning the abdomen and creating a balance between the two brains has already proved useful to patients undergoing radiation or chemotherapy. I see daily evidence of this. My methods have also proved a powerful support tool for those who suffer from the other major scourges of modern society, hypertension and heart disease, and can aid recuperation following surgery or illness.

I firmly believe that maintaining a healthy second brain and encouraging its interaction with the upper brain must be regarded as an invaluable weapon in the fight against medical disorders and innumerable illnesses. It also helps to combat unbalanced states of mind and slow the ageing process. In a nutshell, it's a means of promoting and sustaining good health.

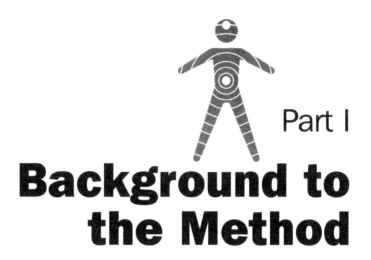

Part I
Background to the Method

My method can be traced back to a childhood that was unremittingly bleak and painful. Today, when I think about those early years, the memory still brings tears to my eyes. My heart contracts. And my stomach hurts.

I was the tenth child in the family. My mother died in childbirth. My father was an upright individual, a disciplinarian perhaps, but not overly strict or pious. He was warm-hearted to a fault, but he was depressed by the injustice of my mother's death and he survived her by only a few years. Together with my brothers, I was placed in a succession of orphanages. We then survived the attentions of self-styled 'caring' families, who seemed to regard the children placed in their charge as little more than additional pairs of hands to help out on the farm.

Looking back, the principal sensation that comes to mind is not one of fear or lack of affection; it is one of hunger. My brothers and I were, to put it bluntly, half-starved. So much so that we used to catch chickens and, fearful of being caught in the act by the gendarmes, pluck them on the spot and eat them raw. Given the opportunity, we were capable of eating our way through an entire crop of strawberries or devouring every single fruit on an apple or pear tree. We also drank litres of milk, which we stole from doorsteps.

As you might expect, this anarchic diet provoked intense stomach cramps on an almost-permanent basis. That is perhaps the abiding childhood memory that still remains vivid to this day. I described this traumatic period in my life at some length in *Le cri du cœur* ('Cry from the Heart'), written in 1996. 'My stomach hurts' was the constant refrain. I was cold. I was sad. I was lonely. But, above all, my stomach hurt.

Looking back today in the light of recent medical research, I am not surprised this was the case. Persistent and at times unbearable stomach pains were clearly attributable to the circumstances to which my brothers and I had fallen victim. Abdominal disorders reflected the anxiety that plagued my second brain. At times, I would literally cry out in pain, and I would resort to the only available 'cure' – lying on my back, knees bent, massaging my stomach. At the time, I had the impression that the warmth from my hands was penetrating the flesh and relieving the immediate anguish. A heated brick or a hot water bottle would doubtless have had the same effect. As a rule, the pain would gradually subside after several minutes and, if I continued rubbing, would eventually ease off entirely. But not for long. At the first sign of anxiety, typically after a slap administered when a mouthful of food was bolted down, the searing pain would start again, spreading inexorably to my back and legs.

At school at Lorgues in the Midi, where I stayed prior to university, I took a succession of part-time jobs to help pay my way, working as a delivery boy, dishwasher, waiter, beach boy, photographer or whatever. I continued to suffer from severe abdominal pain. The agonies persisted into adulthood and were complemented by a series of nervous complaints – lingering depression, rebelliousness and, above all, a persistent feeling of fatigue. I could sense the tension build, and I was afraid it would be with me for the rest of my life.

For a time, I sought solace in sport. Swimming. Running. Cycling. And it seemed to work. I felt better, more balanced. But then the stomach pains reappeared. Today, I understand why: I was pushing myself too hard, punishing my abdomen instead of taking care of it. In effect, the result was the exact opposite of what

I had intended. My problems were compounded by and manifested in recurrent bouts of exhaustion, nervous tension, irritability, sleeplessness and stomach cramps. I had disrupted my natural balance. The stomach pains were still there and, inevitably perhaps, they intensified during my period of military service as a lieutenant in the airborne corps in Algeria. By this time, I had consulted a whole phalanx of gastro-enterologists, ingested a ton of pills and potions, and started to pay attention to my diet. But the problem simply wouldn't go away. I met my future wife on the beach at Cavalaire in the Var region: we married and lived happily ever after – except for one thing: my stomach still played up on a regular basis.

Strangely enough, it was only when I worked with patients that the real dimensions of my own problem gradually became apparent – as did the solution. As luck would have it, I appeared to have inherited something precious from my father – 'good hands', a healing touch, call it what you will. Proof of this emerged while I was working as a beach attendant in Saint-Aygulf. My boss at the time was crippled with lumbago and, one day, I offered to give him a massage. He agreed and I set to work. It wasn't the first time by any means: I'd often practised massage on friends on the farm or at college. Several days later, a gentleman who came to the beach regularly, together with his wife Françoise, also complained of a sore back. My boss suggested I might be able to help. 'Try Pierre,' he said. 'He has a gift for that sort of thing. He certainly worked wonders with my lumbago.'

That patient's name was Pablo Picasso.

Picasso settled on a stool with his heavily muscled back towards me. I positioned myself on a chair behind him and told him to place his hands palms-down on the table in front of him and to rest his head against them. He obeyed, grumbling at the inconvenience of it all. I planted my feet firmly in the sand and started to work on him. Picasso let out the occasional dull groan as I kneaded his spine, but finally started to relax as I put some effort into it. Once I had finished, I did what my father had always done: placed my hands flat against his shoulders and back to disperse the energy field. To my astonishment, I discovered Picasso was sound asleep. Some time later, he invited me to his home in Vallauris, when his back started acting up again. That time – without giving too much thought to it – I also worked on his abdomen.

I planted my feet firmly in the sand and started to work on him. Picasso let out the occasional dull groan as I kneaded his spine, but finally started to relax as I put some effort into it.

I gradually became aware that I did indeed have what people call 'healing hands', and I was determined to use them well. What I noticed time and again was that the typical patient's abdomen was rigid and distended. Even if the patient described his problem as back pain, an aching shoulder, a persistent headache or some other such discomfort, I always made straight for the abdomen, testing it, palpating it, massaging it, first lightly then more intensely, instinctively tracing the contours of the plexus and the meridians. Almost without exception, I could identify some malfunction or other – a temporary malformation, perhaps, or signs of muscle spasm or constipation. And, without further ado, my hands would start working on the abdomen. The results were gratifying and they confirmed that, by focusing on the abdomen, I was also addressing problem areas elsewhere.

When I worked on myself, using a process of self-massage, I experienced the benefits at first hand and I can testify to the effects; in particular, it dissipated the bouts of fatigue that had plagued me in my younger days. Usually, I would lie on my back and, instead of subjecting myself to a gentle massage, I would literally pound my abdomen, pinching and pummelling the skin violently for five or six minutes. The procedure was radical but I still experienced a sense of well-being, as if the pain voluntarily inflicted was somehow mitigating a deeper pain experienced elsewhere.

The interminable stomach pains that once made my life such a misery are now only a vague memory. In time, I found I no longer had to lie on my back, but could massage my abdomen from a sitting position. The physical effort involved was considerable, however, and, in order to relax, I had increasing recourse to deep and regular breathing patterns. This was how I discovered the extraordinary efficacy of massage coupled with proper breathing. My tiredness diminished in spectacular fashion, I started to sleep better, my irritability decreased and my stomach pains were soon fewer and farther between.

Those early experiences proved crucial benchmarks in my development as a therapist. I must admit that as I unlocked the secret of well-being and came to terms with myself and my own body, I became angry at the thought of all that time spent in doctors' surgeries and all the money I had paid for pills of every description. Still, the principal feeling was one of pride. I was no longer a slave to my abdomen. I had learned how to breathe deeply and correctly and I was beginning to appreciate what that implied. I was on the point of developing a method that could have far-reaching implications, namely concentrating treatment on the abdomen as a second brain – a brain with its own peculiar properties and innate characteristics that interfaced with the upper brain.

When, thanks in no small part to my wife Florence, I subsequently started to eat at regular intervals and to eat slowly and without any sense of stress, my pains disappeared for good. It was then that I realised why my patients' abdominal pains seemed to disappear more quickly than my own: on the whole, their lives were less stressful than mine. At the time, I would often rise at four in the morning to make house calls, rush to the hospital where I spent the better part of the day working as a trainee osteopath, then dash off to kinesiology courses given by Boris Dolto[3] before rounding out the day with a further series of evening house calls. I was in perpetual motion, snatching a bite to eat as and when I could. As yet, I remained ignorant of a crucial element in what would later emerge as my method: the need to eat on a regular basis and to eat without undue haste.

I was 28 years old and, although I didn't know it at the time, I had already acquired the key components of what would turn out to be my 'method'. I continued to study and work 'proactively' (as the buzzword goes). I was happy, fit and enthusiastic, and my own complaints were a thing of the past. To my delight, I was able to help a succession of household-name patients – the dress designer Cristóbal Balenciaga, the ballet dancer Rudolf Nureyev, Audrey Hepburn, Ava Gardner, Yul Brynner and Frank Sinatra, authors such as Joseph Kessel, businessman Gianni Agnelli, Princess Grace of Monaco, and presidents and prime ministers throughout the world.

PART I: BACKGROUND TO THE METHOD

I was particularly intrigued by *Les Mains du Miracle* ('Miracle Hands')[4], a book by Joseph Kessel about the life of Heinrich Himmler's masseur, a man called Kersten, who had treated Himmler on an ongoing basis for chronic stomach cramps. At one point in his career, Kersten had the good fortune to meet a Chinese physician named Dr Ko, who had trained in Tibet; he taught Kersten how to locate and manipulate the plexus and the meridians. This was precisely what I had been attempting – intuitively – both on my patients and on myself, albeit with no working knowledge of Chinese medicine. I prevailed upon Hervé Mille, then CEO at *Paris Match*, to introduce me to his good friend Kessel in the hopes of meeting Kersten himself. It was too late: Kersten had died in the interim. When I finally met up with Joseph Kessel, however, he invited me to give him a neck massage (he was experiencing severe headaches at the time) and I duly obliged. Once I had massaged his neck, I made him lie on his back in order to work on his abdomen, which was distended and in spasm. I did my level best to emulate Kersten by vigorously palpating Kessel's plexus and meridians. Kessel groaned as I worked him over. When I finished, he looked at me and said: 'Pierre, you have no cause to envy Kersten. You have the same gift he had.'

That encounter proved a life-changing experience. I knew then that I had a gift, that my hands-on approach genuinely worked. Many of my patients have since expressed astonishment at how beneficial my massage method is and how quickly it achieves results. By working the abdomen, I have achieved positive, even spectacular results, such as improved joint articulation and the alleviation of back pain, fatigue, insomnia and sexual dysfunction – often much to the surprise of my patients' own physicians. In effect, by healing myself, I gained an invaluable insight into how best to create a balance between the two brains. Ever since, I have continued to fine-tune my approach as an integral component of my overriding aim in life: to serve my patients as best as I can.

I took stock. My method had its origins in my childhood and had subsequently been honed by years of study and clinical experience. Ten years studying as an osteopath and dietician had afforded me precious insights into human anatomy, bones and joint structure, cardiac and respiratory systems, and the entire digestive process. I had learned a great deal about nutritional

By working the abdomen, I have achieved positive, even spectacular results, such as improved joint articulation and the alleviation of back pain, fatigue and sexual dysfunction...

values and the consequences of malnutrition and fasting, as well as fad diets. But, despite all this, I was still groping for solutions to abdominal health. Granted, I had practised on patients from every walk of life and had built a sound track record. But there was still something missing. That puzzled me. I cast about for a solution, for some explanation of why the abdomen was so important.

Today, I know why; back then, there was insufficient knowledge about the close interaction between the upper brain and the abdomen, our second brain.

PART I: BACKGROUND TO THE METHOD

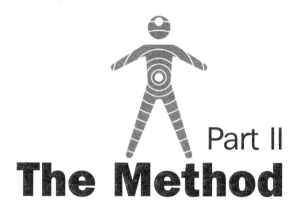

Part II
The Method

THE RULES IN BRIEF

My approach to abdominal health can be broken down into seven constituent elements:

- Abdominal breathing
- Regular and slow eating
- Eating carefully
- Recreational exercise
- Exercises for the two brains
- Self-massage
- Abdominal meditation

Each of these elements is beneficial to overall well-being but in order to address specific disorders, it is essential to follow all of the guidelines. Neglecting one or more will result in less than optimal results.

1. Abdominal Breathing

This is the key to achieving the correct balance between the upper brain and the abdominal second brain. I refer to this as *respiration d'étente-bienêtre*, which roughly translates as 'breathing for relaxation and health'. This is an essential requirement for a healthy abdomen. Once you have acquired – or, to be more exact, *re*-acquired – this breathing technique, you will be astonished at the sustained improvement in your overall well-being.

2. Regular and Slow Eating

In order to function optimally, your abdomen must be nourished in a way that respects your natural biorhythms and prevents any rupture of the link to the upper brain. Regulated and *slow* eating must become a habit – and it should be enjoyed.

3. Eating Carefully

Stop eating whatever comes to hand – and avoid weight-loss diets at all costs. Instead, simply regulate and monitor your food intake with as much care as possible to achieve a balance based on personal preferences, specific health problems and a number of basic guidelines. This is crucial to abdominal health.

4. Recreational Exercise

For the abdomen to function correctly, you need to build strength and endurance through physical exercise. Recreational exercise is important, but some sports are more appropriate than others. I have developed specific guidelines about the form of physical exercise that is best for the body and that will stimulate cardiac and neurological functions while helping mental relaxation.

5. Exercises for the Two Brains

Achieving harmony and balance between the two brains is one of the cornerstones of my method. This means a flat and well-muscled stomach, together with a supple back and joints. I have suggested a number of simple but imaginative 'two-brain' exercises to promote balance on pages 114–19.

6. Self-Massage

To keep your abdomen in optimal shape, it is important to spend a few moments each day on abdominal and head massage. I offer some hints based on my own experience; these are easy to follow and, at the same time, pleasant, relaxing and effective.

7. Abdominal Meditation

It has been demonstrated that the abdomen is not merely an inert collection of tubes but rather an autonomous cellular organ intimately linked to the upper brain. I invite you to start 'thinking' about and *with* your abdomen and to understand its contribution to sustained health and well-being.

The seven guidelines described above are discussed in greater detail in the following pages.

Note: When practising exercises the following scale is useful:

●   = easy
●●   = slightly more difficult
●●●   = moderately difficult
●●●● = requires concentration/difficult

PART II: THE METHOD

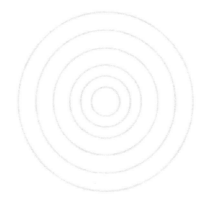

ABDOMINAL BREATHING

THE PLAIN FACT OF THE MATTER is that most people do not breathe correctly. The majority of adults and, without exception, every adolescent I encounter in the course of my daily practice breathes to only about 50 per cent of their capacity.

Social pressures are to blame for this loss of natural breathing capacity. In early childhood, up to the age of two years or so, when consciousness of 'self' and the external world begins to manifest itself, children fill their lungs and abdomen with air – and empty both in a similar fashion. Later, when the pressures of the outside world come into play – introducing emotions such as stress, anxiety, timidity – the respiratory rhythm accelerates and the initial, natural and spontaneous practice of deep breathing gives way to 'social' breathing, which is less deep and confined to the lungs and the bronchial tubes (and, even there, is only partial). As a result, the volume of air ingested into the body is reduced by approximately half.

We have become accustomed to not breathing with our abdomen. For several reasons, this is nothing short of catastrophic.

First and foremost, it is catastrophic for the abdomen itself. When it doesn't get enough oxygen, the abdomen becomes sluggish and underperforms. This invites the onset of disorders such as colitis, constipation and stomach cramps. Problems absorbing food and eliminating waste materials lead to exhaustion, insomnia, nervous tension, weight gain, sexual dysfunction, allergies and many other debilitating conditions.[5]

In my view, there are even more serious consequences. By abandoning the practice of abdominal breathing that we followed spontaneously in our early years, we unwittingly sever the link between the second and first brains and provoke other disorders in addition to compounding those noted above. If the 'upper' and 'lower' brains are not in tune, no amount of anti-depressants or anxiolytic (anxiety-reducing) drugs will be sufficient to induce the state of relaxation that is fundamental to overall well-being.

Men and women have different breathing patterns. In men, breathing tends to be from the diaphragm, whereas in women it is costal (in the ribs) and thoracic (in the chest). However, under stress, men and women tend to lapse into the same breathing patterns. Roughly speaking, inhalation takes something over a second, and exhalation the same. In other words, we inhale and exhale some 20 times a minute, or 1,200 times every hour, and around 15,000 times a day, with allowance made for slower breathing patterns during non-waking hours. I once calculated that on an annual basis, the typical human inhales and exhales roughly 5.5 million times. Breathing imparts a natural rhythm to our lives and is a precondition of survival. By re-oxygenating the blood, we keep our vital organs functioning, not least the two most vital organs of all, the abdomen and the upper brain.

The daily pressures of modern life impact negatively on our breathing patterns. Sedentary lifestyles and junk food exacerbate the problem. On the whole, we breathe more rapidly and less fully today than we did 20 or 30 years ago.

Take the case of Emmanuelle: 27 years old, single, pretty, a senior management employee. She sleeps intermittently, if at all. She complains of periods of emotional stress punctuated by

The daily pressures of modern life impact negatively on our breathing patterns. Sedentary lifestyles and junk food exacerbate the problem.

bouts of depression. Her emotional life is a roller-coaster. Twice a week, she attends an aerobics class and she also works out in the gym. She is convinced that physical exercise will help her relax, overcome her feelings of anxiety and, not least, help her sleep better. She describes herself as 'choosy' as far as food is concerned, but she eats quickly and drinks three or four cups of coffee daily as well as that all-important first cup, without which (she insists) she simply cannot function.

An initial examination reveals a well-toned body. But her abdomen is tight, cramped and painfully distended. It is immediately evident that Emmanuelle's exercise routine is too rigorous and that she works out too late in the day, with the result that her biological rhythms are out of synch and her feeling of exhaustion is intensified. I try to explain to her that, believe it or not, we should be preparing for bed at five in the afternoon and that, instead of a vigorous workout, she should consider a more gentle and relaxing form of exercise. At the same time, I convince her to stop drinking coffee (although an exception may be made for the early-morning cup, providing she eats something solid beforehand). She also agrees to take time over her meals. Not least, Emmanuelle assures me she will practise my 'breathe-to-relax' method once every hour.

Three weeks later, Emmanuelle is a different person. Her abdomen is supple and relaxed. The stress lines on her face have vanished. She is sleeping well. The new abdominal breathing technique has benefited her entire body, with every organ and gland deriving maximum benefit from an increased oxygen intake.

This case study demonstrates my view that abdominal breathing is the first step on the road to full health. And, once again, it is a matter of achieving a proper balance between the two brains.

Centre Stage for the Abdomen

My initial approach consists of teaching patients to re-learn how to breathe from the abdomen as naturally and as instinctively as they did in early childhood. The procedure is not difficult or unduly onerous but, once you have mastered it – in a matter of days or, at worst, after two weeks – you will immediately feel the benefits, both physical and mental. You'll feel a sense of relaxation almost immediately, which is a clear indication that your two brains are beginning to work in tandem and that, as a result, your entire body is more 'in tune'.

The first step is to understand that you must breathe into your abdomen if that organ is to regain the primary function it served in early childhood. Grasping that simple notion will help you follow the simple procedures outlined below.

The initial objective is to unblock the diaphragm, the powerful muscle located between the chest and the abdomen, below the heart and above the digestive tract. The diaphragm is the key instrument used to produce deep breathing. It is constantly active, rising and falling some 20 times a minute as you breathe in and out. The amplitude of this up-and-down movement determines not only the amount of air absorbed into the system but

All it takes is an additional one-and-a-half seconds of inhalation for the upper brain to increase its output of endorphins, which help us to combat stress and external threats.

also the overall functioning of the abdomen.

Abdominal breathing patterns provide a natural massage for vital organs such as the gall bladder, the liver, the pancreas, the spleen and the intestines, as well as facilitating the digestive processes of absorption and elimination. What is more, by stimulating the plexus – which is directly linked to the upper brain via the vagus nerve (see box) – harmony between the two brains is reinforced. When the pituitary gland situated at the base of the skull is fed an improved supply of oxygen, it generates additional endorphins (pain inhibitors), which are often referred to as 'health hormones'. All it takes is an additional one-and-a-half seconds of inhalation for the upper brain to increase its output

Breathing and the Vagus Nerve

Our two brains communicate via an intermediary known as the vagus nerve, or the pneumo-gastric nerve. This runs from the skull down the neck, across the chest and into the abdomen, transiting the cardiovascular, respiratory and digestive systems and supplying organs and glands.

In the respiratory system, the vagus nerve stimulates the production of mucus in the respiratory tract (pharynx, larynx, oesophagus, trachea, lungs and bronchia) and dictates the rhythm, frequency and intensity of breathing patterns.[6] Thanks to the vagus nerve, each breathing phase, irrespective of its intensity, is simultaneously 'registered' by both the upper and lower brains.

of endorphins, which help us to combat stress and external threats. Endorphins help various anatomical systems to function more effectively and when more of them are released, the development of immune cells in the abdomen is stimulated.

It is not difficult to learn to breathe more deeply and more slowly. From time to time we all need to accelerate our breathing and to breathe more deeply, notably during strenuous physical effort or in response to stress, when the body clamours for more oxygen. All that is required is to use your abdomen to breathe more slowly and more deeply on a regular rather than on an exceptional basis.

It is important to free up your diaphragm. Typically it will

PART II: THE METHOD

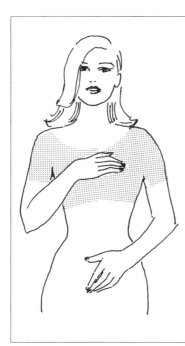

Learning abdominal breathing

Breathing air into the abdomen does not take strenuous effort, merely a bit of concentration. As you breathe, place a hand on your stomach; you will feel it expand and contract. Early on, this movement will be virtually imperceptible, but it will soon become more pronounced. You will also notice that, at the same time as your chest inflates and deflates, your abdomen will rise and fall accordingly. The movement is less pronounced in the chest, but it will also be felt. You will soon realise that you have acquired the ability to breathe abdominally. And your life will never be the same again.

have a tendency to 'block' in response to more precipitate and shorter breathing patterns. To free it, try imagining that the air you inhale is destined in the first instance for your abdomen. You may find it tricky but once you have mastered the technique, you will quickly experience the benefits.

Secrets of Abdominal Breathing

Start by practising abdominal breathing while lying down; later, the inhale-exhale manoeuvre involving lungs and abdomen can be practised in any position you choose – seated, upright, standing still or moving. The process will soon become second nature once your abdomen is 'liberated' and schooled to accept and expel the air you send to it.

This in-out breathing pattern (described in detail on pages 46–8) should be practised five times every hour. It must be stressed yet again that this is the cornerstone of my method. In other words, advice given elsewhere in this book regarding nutrition, exercise, meditation, two-brain balance and so on, is conditional upon mastering abdominal breathing.

Once you have 'liberated' your diaphragm, you will find you have more control over it and are able to breathe more slowly and more deeply, thereby contributing to abdominal health and a sense of overall well-being. An immediate benefit will be increased protection against outside stressors, lapses in

By following this in-out breathing technique 40 to 50 times a day, you will have oxygenated your system and stimulated your blood flow by the same amount as if you had completed a 10-kilometre (6-mile) walk!

concentration and even poor eating habits. By practising five times an hour, you will begin to feel calmer and more relaxed as your two brains gradually achieve optimal harmony.

You can practise wherever you are – at home, at work, in the car or on public transport. You may initially experience a feeling of dizziness, even a touch of vertigo. This is not a cause for concern: it is attributable to your increased oxygen intake, which may temporarily accelerate the heart rate. By following this in-out breathing technique 40 to 50 times a day, you will have oxygenated your system and stimulated your blood flow by the same amount as if you had completed a 10-kilometre (6-mile) walk! If by some chance you should experience any other symptoms, all you need to do is cut back to three times hourly. When the symptoms recede, you can then return to the five-times-an-hour cycle.

I am convinced you will very quickly identify beneficial effects after following my abdominal breathing method. These benefits will not be confined to the abdomen; other glands and organs are naturally massaged by the increased movement of the diaphragm. Over the years, I have noted the extent to which a return to the abdominal breathing patterns of early childhood are accompanied by a whole series of physical benefits, including improved blood supply to the intestinal tract, a key factor in the absorption of nutrients and the elimination of waste products. Abdominal breathing is one of the key principles of yoga.

I recently came across some studies by Dr John Seskevitch of the University of North Carolina who, over the past 15 years or so, has taught abdominal breathing techniques to no fewer than 18,000 patients, approximately half of whom were cancer sufferers. I quote:

I do not pretend to have cured them by virtue of abdominal respiration techniques, but I have witnessed significant improvement in their condition and considerably reduced their time spent in intensive care units. This was especially true of patients who, for years, had repeatedly been told simply to 'relax'. Abdominal breathing proved useful in stimulating the oxygenation process in the case of those with respiratory disorders and I was able to report a favourable impact on their overall condition.[7]

A Harmonious Relationship

Breathing is the only physiological function that can be consciously activated. It is governed in part by the nervous system (by the vagus, cranial and certain spinal nerves) and it can be influenced by emotions or mental or physical exertion, but respiration can also be activated, accelerated or decelerated by a conscious effort of will. In other words, we are capable of modifying its amplitude and rhythm, even to the point of shutting it down – at least, until the point where the body, deprived of oxygen, automatically kicks back in to avoid suffocation.

It's in our best interests to take advantage of this control but I don't recommend going as far as those yogi who, by controlling their breathing, can effectively reduce their body temperature and blood pressure to the point of suppressing all sensation. I do recommend that you take the fullest possible advantage of your new-found natural breathing ability. Learning to breathe correctly is rejuvenating, as any opera singer can confirm.

Once you have mastered the technique of inflating and emptying your abdomen at the same time as your lungs, you will impart new life and vibrancy to your abdomen and help it fulfil its role as your second brain. The link between this second brain and the upper brain – and I cannot emphasise this too much – is an essential component of a healthy lifestyle and an invaluable tool in warding off all manner of complaints and disorders. Where this two-brain harmony is not in place, the abdomen cannot function as it should. By the same token, a healthy abdomen is a precondition of the optimal functioning of the upper brain, which is the seat of our senses, intelligence, intuition and emotions.

Re-Learning to Breathe through the Abdomen

Exercise 1

Lie flat on your back, legs bent, and place one book on your stomach and another on your chest. Place a hand on each book, breathe in gently through the nose for seven to ten seconds and attempt to direct the air intake towards your abdomen. You may find this difficult at first because your abdomen is no longer in the habit of taking in air or responding to the 'inhale-exhale' signal sent by the upper brain. The abdomen can be 'blocked', in which case your breathing patterns are dominated by the chest. Keep trying and don't be discouraged. It will work. After a few attempts, you will feel the book placed on your stomach start to rise and fall, almost imperceptibly at first (see diagram A). Congratulations! You have re-learned how to breathe abdominally.

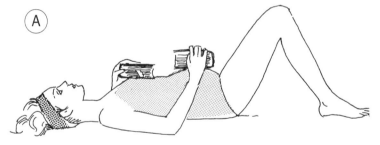

You will notice that, as you inhale and exhale, the book on your chest will rise and fall in the same rhythm as that on your stomach. This means that you are breathing 'globally', that the link between your two brains has been re-established, and that you are poised to reap the benefits described earlier.

Pause for a second or two between inhalation and exhalation by retaining the air in your lungs and abdomen. Then exhale through the nose or mouth, trying to empty the abdomen first

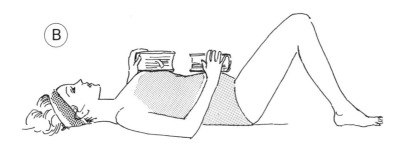

(the book placed there will descend slowly, see diagram B) and then the lungs. When you have completely exhaled, pull in your stomach as far as possible (imagine bringing your navel towards your spinal column). The exhalation phase should also take between seven and ten seconds, after which time both books will have descended significantly.

Exercise 2

Sit on a chair or stool and place both hands on your abdomen. Breathe in slowly through the nose for seven to ten seconds, then direct the inhaled air towards the abdomen, inflating it (see diagram A). Pause for one or two seconds before exhaling for seven to ten seconds, at the same time pressing your clenched fists against the abdomen to deflate it as far as possible (see diagram B, over).

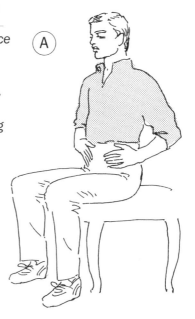

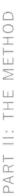

PART II: THE METHOD

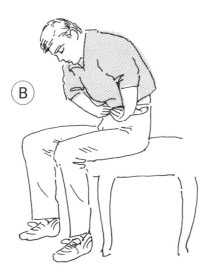

In the unlikely event that you can't unblock your diaphragm and force air into the abdomen, consult a therapist or, if you have a friend who is a professional athlete, actor, singer or musician, try discussing it with them. They should be familiar with abdominal breathing techniques as a matter of course.

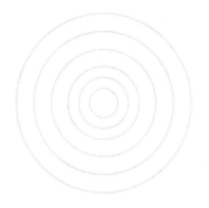

REGULAR AND SLOW EATING

LIKE THE UPPER BRAIN, THE ABDOMEN is constantly active, day in, day out. Cerebral processes do not shut down at night: we dream. Equally, abdominal processes remain active: the processes of digestion, absorption and elimination are uninterrupted through the night.

Optimal abdominal health is to a large degree governed by what we eat, although other factors enter into the complex equation. As a practitioner treating abdominal problems, I am aware of the abdomen's innate properties as a preventive and restorative organ and convinced of the importance of what we eat and how we eat it.

Eating is both a necessity and a pleasure. Typically, a 60-year-old will have devoted more than five years of his or her life to ingesting food. Some cynics might argue that eating and drinking are merely signposts along the road to death, but I take the opposite view: I believe that what we eat and drink is what helps us remain healthy. Provided, that is, that we do not eat indiscriminately (there's more about this on pages 61–9).[8]

Perhaps the first point to be made is that when we eat is of critical importance. Eating 'on the run' or as the opportunity presents itself is simply not good enough. Although we have gained substantial insight into the functioning of the upper brain – discovering, for example, that the regenerative powers of sleep are more pronounced in the initial rather than in the later hours, or that dreams recur in cycles – we are still not totally sure how our 'second' brain processes food, despite the fact that this is crucial to the overall well-being of the abdomen.

Respect Your Body Clock

Our lives are regulated from infancy onwards by what is commonly referred to as a body clock, for which the secret mechanism is located in the hypothalamus. Among other things, it controls 'automatic' functions such as body temperature and hunger. Our body clock is central to our general health, not least the digestive processes performed by the abdomen. When it comes to nutrition, we ignore those natural rhythms at our peril.

In days gone by, mealtimes were sacred and hallowed by observance – particularly in rural areas, where falling ill was simply not an option. I recall from my own childhood how fieldworkers would simply not tolerate any departure from the time-honoured rituals of a punctual breakfast and midday meal. Staying healthy was a precondition of running a farm and tending to crops and livestock. Mealtimes were set and respected back then, when labour laws were fluid and statutory maximum working hours simply unheard of.

Times have changed. Today, we tend to eat what we like, as and when we choose, and whenever time permits. To my mind, the consequences of this have proved disastrous. Once our body clock has been tampered with and abused, the system fights back. The digestive cycle is disrupted at the level of the solar plexus, the gall bladder, the pancreas and the intestine, triggering a destabilisation of the tenuous relationship between the two brains. Once that balance is upset, internal rhythms are thrown into disarray. Systems malfunction and serious illnesses may result, including

> **Today, we tend to eat what we like, as and when we choose, and whenever time permits. To my mind, the consequences of this have proved disastrous.**

the onset of allergies, depleted energy levels and a higher incidence of heart problems.

I recall the case of Simone S., a 42-year-old divorcee who lived alone following the collapse of her marriage. She ate sporadically and haphazardly, irrespective of whether she was hungry. She did not derive any pleasure from what she ate. Worse, she put on 12 kilos (26 lbs) and, partly as a result, her self-confidence was eroded. She experimented with various diets, but they appeared only to make matters worse.

I persuaded Simone that a first priority was to re-set her body clock. By adopting my breathe-to-relax approach and keeping a personal 'food journal' (see pages 68–9), she was able to track the shortcomings in her behaviour. During the first week of eating more slowly and at specified times, she lost 2 kilos (4 lbs). Her abdomen became less distended and less prone to cramps. This convinced her to persist with my method and to take up regular physical exercise, abdominal meditation and my other recommendations. Simone's two brains were eventually reconciled. She lost a further 10 kilos (22 lbs) of unwanted weight, slimmed down to her pre-divorce figure, became progressively more self-confident and regained a happy (and healthy) outlook on life generally.

Simone's experience demonstrates the importance of eating regularly to maintain good natural biorhythms, as well as the need for a sustained link between the abdomen and the upper brain as a barrier against digestive system dysfunction. In practice, this may mean eating three, four or even five meals a day, depending on your occupation or level of activity. 'Hunger' – the appetite engendered simultaneously by the two brains – will be the decisive factor in setting your individual body clock.[9] Above all, remember that a chaotic and intermittent approach to eating is totally incompatible with a healthy abdomen.

There will always be situations where disruption of the body clock is unavoidable; for example, when working on night shifts or travelling on long-haul flights. Several recent studies have examined the effects of such disruption[10], while others have looked at the consequences of eating and drinking late at night.[11] It transpires that the latter may well induce a rise in cholesterol levels, more fatty deposits in the arteries and a whole host of other negative symptoms that could culminate in diabetes or other serious disorders. The digestive process works more slowly at night than during the day, so a meal taken around midnight will produce higher blood sugar levels than the same meal eaten at midday.

If a meal is eaten very quickly or under stressful conditions, the damage can be considerable. One immediate consequence of eating a meal too quickly is the more rapid onset of the desire to smoke or consume harmful stimulants such as coffee, tea or alcohol. As is well known, these can lead to coronaries, allergies and a reduction in overall energy.

Researchers have also looked long and hard at the practice of fasting, often as a religious observance (for example during Ramadan)[12], and have noted chemical, physical and even hormonal changes that occur as a result. Personally, I am against fasting in any form, since I regard it as shirking our responsibilities to our bodies. Equally, I always counsel against skipping a meal; my preference in the event of 'not feeling hungry' would be to eat at the regular time but simply reduce the quantity of food ingested. If you are ill or otherwise under the weather, it is even more inadvisable to skip meals and risk re-setting your body clock.

I also strongly advise against weight-loss programmes or diets designed to alleviate specific complaints. Depriving the organism of essential vitamins can prove injurious to health by weakening the immune defences after a period as short as four days (as clinical tests have demonstrated[13]). In effect, the stomach secretes gastric juices at regular intervals in a process known as chronobiology (the biology of cyclical physiological phenomena); accordingly, if those juices have little or nothing to work on, they convert into acids and other toxins which contaminate the entire digestive system and provoke disorders such as fatigue, weight gain, rheumatism and assorted other disorders. If your body clock is re-set for some reason or other – typically

Bulimia, Snacking and Hunger Pangs

Bulimia is the term applied to a compulsive desire to eat even when not hungry and, worse, to eat anything and everything at any time of day or night. The condition comes about as the result of an imbalance between the two brains. Without exception, bulimia induces an excessive accumulation of fat.

Snacking is a colloquial term, which refers to the repeated and automatic ingestion of small quantities of food. Snacking is not always provoked by hunger and its principal effect is the production of a blood sugar 'high' and a surfeit of insulin, while fatty acids accumulate and are dispersed more slowly. Cravings will return as soon as blood sugar subsides.

Hunger pangs are an urgent need to eat between meals. The cause may be that the preceding meal was inadequate, but they may be a result of hypoglycaemia, an abnormally low concentration of sugar in the blood brought on, for example, by sustained physical exertion or emotional shock.

Bulimia, snacking and hunger pains disrupt the proper functioning of the digestive system, causing it to malfunction or underperform. This, in turn, induces blockages in the liver, pancreas and bile ducts. The consequences range from chronic indigestion to distension of the colon and intestines and inflammation of the intestinal membrane. There are rapid swings in body weight, which affect the blood sugar level, prompting tiredness, nervous depression, cardiovascular, lymphatic and hormonal disorders and a destabilisation of the balance between the abdomen and the upper brain.

by eating at odd hours, 'snacking' or raiding the 'fridge during the night – you must take whatever steps are necessary to get it back on track.

Our stomachs are programmed to to break down fats during the night (a process known as 'nocturnal lipolysis'). To kick-start the system the following morning, it is best to start with a light breakfast (see pages 94–5), then allow a four-hour interval between subsequent meals. After several days, your body clock will re-establish its natural rhythm and will function in accord with your neurological and hormonal cycles again.

Relaxation

Two basic rules govern the method I have developed to help promote abdominal health: first, eat at regular intervals; second, eat when you are relaxed. The second stipulation warrants closer inspection.

Stress and related emotional factors such as anxiety and irritability disrupt the natural cycle of absorption and elimination. These factors may induce the abdomen to start secreting excessive quantities of undesirable acids; equally, the gall-bladder may secrete too much or too little bile and the pancreas may over-produce insulin, leading to familiar conditions such as heartburn, cramps, cold sweats or disorders further down in the intestine and colon. The pylorus, or sphincter muscle, located between the stomach and the duodenum, is particularly sensitive to stress, agitation or the ingestion of stimulants such as coffee, alcohol or tobacco. The sphincter muscle opens once the mass of chewed

Continued on page 58

PART II: THE METHOD

Intestinal Flora

The digestive tract in a new-born infant is sterile. Colonies of bacteria begin to form there after 48 hours or so, their specific composition dictated by whether the baby is breast- or bottle-fed. Between the ages of three and six months, intestinal flora mutate to generate antibodies and, by the age of five years, the body's immune system is fully matured. (The term 'intestinal micro-flora' describes some 100,000 *billion* bacteria from approximately four hundred different strains.)

Stress and anxiety rapidly affect the digestive process by stimulating or decelerating intestinal activity and modifying these micro-flora. In the event of abdominal malfunction, the inherent advantages of micro-flora are dissipated. These advantages include[14]:

- countering the build-up of fatty acids, thereby decreasing harmful ('bad') cholesterol
- breaking down any nutrients that are not absorbed by the small intestine
- helping vitamins to be absorbed by the action of 'good' bacteria
- eliminating or suppressing pathogenic bacteria
- protecting against hypersensitivity, inflammation and allergies; and
- reinforcing the intestinal immune system.

Certain foods, notably fruit, vegetables and tea, contain fibres and antioxidants that are resistant to digestive enzymes; these are particularly beneficial for modifying and reinforcing intestinal flora. Needless to say, a healthy abdomen, with a fully functional defence network of intestinal flora, is essential to combat the stresses and strains of modern life.

Research shows that stress at mealtimes reduces the secretion of cortisone, melatonin and testosterone, among other substances. Even eating while watching television can harm the digestive system. When emotional stress is registered by the upper brain – perhaps while watching news reports of a violent nature – it provokes micro-traumas in the second brain, the abdomen. The rapidly changing images, colours and light levels can also be harmful. For these reasons, I categorically stipulate that meals should not be eaten on your lap before the TV set but at the dining table. I also insist that, if you have been and/or remain stressed by the events of the day, my recommended exercises for healthy breathing (see pages 36–48) should precede a meal.

Relaxing at mealtimes helps to restore the balance between the two brains, whereby the upper brain assumes responsibility for nurturing abdominal receptivity. I always advise my patients to follow some kind of routine at mealtimes, perhaps rotating the tasks of serving the meal and clearing up afterwards. I am also convinced that a short walk after a meal or even simply washing up is conducive to relaxation and proper digestion.

PART II: THE METHOD

food (known as the alimentary bolus) has been properly processed in the stomach. Approximately 90 minutes after food is eaten, the bolus is passed through the sphincter in measured quantities of appropriate consistency. The sphincter is like a customs official at a border control, in that it monitors the passage of chewed food into the lower intestine, ensures the build-up of benign intestinal flora (see box, pages 56–7), and regulates the entire digestive process, protecting against cramps, fermentation, distension, chronic indigestion, constipation and other undesirable conditions. Blockage of the sphincter – which is directly connected to the upper brain – may provoke vomiting.

The sphincter is like a customs official at a border control, in that it monitors the passage of chewed food into the lower intestine… and regulates the entire digestive process…

The above digestive complaints are registered by the upper brain and can cause periods of irritability and anxiety, or lassitude and diminished concentration.

Eating Slowly

Another major element in my method is an insistence on eating *slowly*. This is one of the prerequisites of second-brain health.

Never – ever – eat quickly and without chewing your food properly. From the very first mouthful, you should be salivating. Saliva is a mixture of water, proteins and mineral salts (calcium, phosphorus) which helps to protect the teeth and, thanks to its enzymes, reduces oral acidity. Its disinfectant properties are of vital importance in the absorption–elimination process.

It is essential to realise that the digestive process begins before you start eating when you feel your mouth watering. In the total or partial absence of saliva, several problems arise, among them that of excess gastric acid. Coffee, tea, tobacco and alcohol ingested on an empty stomach are all 'destabilisers' that affect the gastric juices, while nerve-depressants and anti-inflammatory medication can provoke digestive disorders and dysfunctions, or cause unwanted weight gain. All medications, except homeopathic ones, may alter the composition of saliva, causing a dry mouth; in addition to imparting a different taste to your food, such drugs can also harm the abdomen.

It was with the above in mind that I developed a series of exercises to 'self-massage' the face and skull and stimulate the nerve endings that are attached to the vagus. Self-massage not only increases saliva secretion, but it also relaxes the central nervous system; as a result, the technique affects the sensations of taste, smell, sight and hearing. Stimulating sensitive sites on the face also aids the process of digestion. Try self-massage whenever you find yourself producing too little saliva or when you are taking medication. My recommended breathe-to-relax exercises (see pages 46–8) also promote the secretion of saliva.

We are still some way from a full understanding of the role of saliva in the digestive process. Several research laboratories have already invested huge sums trying to develop synthetic saliva and such a breakthrough would doubtless have beneficial effects for abdominal health generally. On the other hand, it's debatable whether the unique properties of saliva can ever be successfully replicated synthetically, bearing in mind that it generates spon-

PART II: THE METHOD

Self-Massaging the Face and Head

Massage your jaws with the tips of your fingers, exerting extra pressure on any painful areas. Work each point for several seconds using a circular motion. Then move your fingers along the nose, around the eyes and across the eyebrows, focusing on the site of the ophthalmic

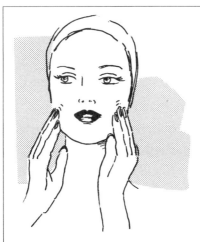

nerve at the point where the inside of the eye meets the top of the nose. Finally, massage your temples and your forehead, working gradually back to the crown of the head. Be careful to avoid any movement that creates friction.

This massage technique invigorates the salivary glands, and it also stimulates the cranial nerve endings so it works positively on the vagus nerve that links the two brains.

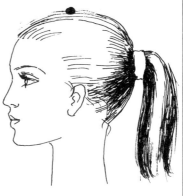

taneously within a fraction of a second in response to an emotion transmitted by the upper brain.

Eating slowly is vital, but even that is not enough. Good oral hygiene is a must. A tooth infection can upset the fragile chemical balance of saliva, with serious consequences for the digestive process as a whole. I have frequently encountered cases where digestive disorders have vanished without trace following a course of dental treatment.

Logging Your Daily Food Intake

Maintaining a healthy link between your abdomen and the upper brain is dependent on the types of food and drink you ingest on a day-to-day basis, the number of meals you eat and their duration. Bear in mind that, just as we all boast a unique set of fingerprints, we also exhibit a unique approach to eating. To understand yours, you should monitor your intake of food and drink closely.

Nothing could be more simple. Buy a little notebook and carry it with you at all times. Note down everything you eat, together with the physical and mental state each food induces. After no more than a week, you will identify patterns and practices that have gone unsuspected sometimes for years on end. After that first 'trial' week, you should start modifying your eating habits and, by the end of week four, you should have dealt with any shortcomings in your diet. From that point onwards, you will begin to experience the positive effects of my method in terms of abdominal health and the well-being of your central nervous system. You will have graduated as your own personal dietician! A number of points should be borne in mind when compiling your journal:

Number of Meals Ideally, you should eat three times a day, including a mandatory breakfast. Depending on your occupation (manual or otherwise), you may add a mid-morning 'treat' and/or some form of mid-afternoon refreshment. On no account, however, may you snack continuously throughout the day.

Mealtimes In principle, there should be a minimum of four hours between each meal, but this can be reduced to three if your occupation involves intense physical or intellectual effort.

Eating Mode You must be relaxed prior to and during eating. You must eat sitting down and in peaceful surroundings, as ambient noise has a negative effect on digestion.

Speed You must eat slowly in order to stimulate the absorption–elimination process and to ensure that your food is properly salivated.

Eating for Pleasure What you eat must reflect your personal preference and appetite. Remember to keep your diet varied.

Smoking Tobacco and vitamins are sworn enemies. Smoking one cigarette kills all the vitamins present in your body at the time. Never smoke at table. Each cigarette shortens life expectancy by an estimated twelve minutes. Feel free to do the sums yourself.

Stress If you feel stressed before a meal, practise my abdominal breathing technique and wait until you feel calmer.

The Ideal Menu This should include the three categories of food: carbohydrates, proteins and fats, plus vitamins and trace elements; the menu should be varied from one meal to the next.

Liquids Avoid sugary drinks at all costs. Have at most one glass of wine or beer, ideally halfway through the meal. Drink still mineral water, varying the brand.

Immediately After a Meal... you should feel well, rested, relaxed and ready to face the world.

... and One to Three Hours Later Pay careful attention to your digestion. Note any foodstuffs that cause physical discomfort (heartburn, wind, cramps, bloating, drowsiness) or a psychological reaction (lapses in concentration, or anxiety). Do not eliminate an individual product; simply reduce its quantity or reverse the sequence of courses. For example, melon or tomato may not agree with you as a starter, but may be more readily digested as a dessert. Equally, eating a whole artichoke may cause wind, but eating only half may be perfectly acceptable. Raw vegetables are more readily digested at the beginning of a meal than at the end. Remember to reduce quantities of sweet desserts, as sugar retards the digestive process.

On the following pages you will see the 'Dos' and 'Don'ts' of eating to keep your abdomen healthy. Using the Personal Planner on pages 68–9 you will be able to record your own eating habits and assess the changes you need to make to achieve optimal abdominal health and well-being.

PART II: THE METHOD

KEEPING YOUR ABDOMEN HEALTHY: DOs and DON'Ts

What NOT to Do...

The following table relates to a typical day in the life of a man or woman working outdoors. Their eating patterns should be

Note the food and drink consumed and the conditions under which they were eaten or drunk			
	Breakfast	**Snack**	**Lunch**
Time	08.00	10.00	13.00
Fast or Slow?	Fast	Fast	Fast
Enjoyed? (Yes or No)	No	No	No
Hungry? (Yes or No)	No	No	No
Smoking? (Yes or No)	No	Yes	Yes
Surroundings (Restful or Noisy)	Restful	Restful	Noisy
Seated or Standing?	Standing	Standing	Seated
Relaxed or Stressed?	Stressed	Stressed	Stressed
Food	Croissant		Mixed salad; steak + fries: apple tart
Drinks	Coffee (black)	Coffee (black)	Wine (2 glasses); coffee (black)

revised if they want to maintain a healthy abdomen and stave off illness.

Snack	Dinner	'Nibbles' (day)	'Nibbles' (night)
	20.00	09.00	
	Slow	Fast	
	Yes	No	
	Yes	No	
	Yes	Yes	
	Restful	Restful	
	Seated + TV	Standing	
	Relaxed	Stressed	
	Soup; fish fillet; rice; caramel pudding	Chocolate bar	Dry biscuits
	Apéritif; wine (2 glasses)	Coffee (black)	Fizzy drink

KEEPING YOUR ABDOMEN HEALTHY: DOs and DON'Ts

What to DO...

The following table relates to a typical day in the life of a man

Note the food and drink consumed and the conditions under which they were eaten or drunk			
	Breakfast	*Snack*	*Lunch*
Time	07.00	10.00	13.00
Fast or Slow?	Slow	Slow	Slow
Enjoyed? (Yes or No)	Yes	Yes	Yes
Hungry? (Yes or No)	Yes	Yes	Yes
Smoking? (Yes or No)	No	No	No
Surroundings (Restful or Noisy)	Restful	Restful	Restful
Seated or Standing?	Seated	Seated	Seated
Relaxed or Stressed?	Relaxed	Relaxed	Relaxed
Food	Light (see pages 94–5)	Fresh fruit	Grilled chicken; rice; fruit salad
Drinks	Weak tea	Mineral water	Wine (1 glass); mineral water; coffee

or woman working outdoors. Their eating patterns are consistent with my method.

Snack	Dinner	'Nibbles' (day)	'Nibbles' (night)
16.00	20.00		
Slow	Slow		
Yes	Yes		
Yes	Yes		
No	No		
Restful	Restful		
Seated	Seated		
Relaxed	Relaxed		
Square of chocolate; slice of wholemeal bread	Salad; grilled sole; spinach; natural yoghurt		
Mineral water	Wine (1 glass); mineral water		

KEEPING YOUR ABDOMEN HEALTHY: DOs and DON'Ts

Personal Planner

Photocopy the following table and use it to record your own eating habits.

Note the food and drink consumed and the conditions under which they were eaten or drunk			
	Breakfast	**Snack**	**Lunch**
Time			
Fast or Slow?			
Enjoyed? (Yes or No)			
Hungry? (Yes or No)			
Smoking? (Yes or No)			
Surroundings (Restful or Noisy)			
Seated or Standing?			
Relaxed or Stressed?			
Food			
Drinks			

Snack	Dinner	'Nibbles' (day)	'Nibbles' (night)

PART II: THE METHOD

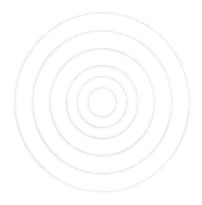

EATING CAREFULLY

IT CAME AS NO GREAT SURPRISE to me when scientific research finally proved the interaction between the abdomen and the upper brain via a complex network of neuro-transmitters. I had long since reached the same conclusion.

I had never been in doubt that strong emotions, a sudden shock or an attack of nerves experienced in the upper brain would affect the abdomen; that the process worked in the other direction, however, was nothing short of a breakthrough in medical science. It was now clear that an abdominal disorder that causes a malfunction of the absorption–elimination process influences the upper brain as well and may be the source of more serious complaints.

An extremely complex and highly diversified network of neuro-transmitters has been discovered, and their full extent and implications have yet to be explored. We already know that messages are carried between the two brains by neuro-transmitters such as serotonin and noradrenaline, which are secreted by the upper brain, but there is every reason to believe that an unknown number of other neuro-transmitters may be involved as well. By the same token, we now know that the majority of the body's immune cells (which ensure protection against harmful bacteria and viruses) are generated in the abdomen. Two-way co-ordination between the two brains is a fact of life, which is now recognised as being of increasing relevance and importance.

One immediate consequence of recent research relates to our diet, which is now recognised as being of crucial relevance to our quest for 'health' and 'well-being', a precondition of overall 'happiness'. My years spent treating the abdomen, massaging it to relieve knots, cramps and even partial or total paralysis induced by stress, have not been wasted. I have successfully treated a whole range of debilitating complaints and disorders, including back pain, fatigue, insomnia, rheumatism, allergies, sexual dysfunction and many other illnesses. By working closely with my medical colleagues, I have also been able to help cure more serious conditions such as type 2 diabetes, cardiac problems and nervous disorders.[15] I have even contributed to the successful treatment of carcinogenic tumours by providing complementary therapy. That my instinctive approach and methodology have now been 'scientifically' vindicated is not only gratifying, but also attests to the importance I have always attached to a healthy abdomen and proper eating patterns as key constituents of a balanced lifestyle.

The importance of the third pillar of my method (after abdominal breathing and regular and slow eating), namely the selection of foods and drinks, has also been vindicated.

PART II: THE METHOD

We Are What We Eat

'We are what we eat' has become something of cliché these days, with good reason. Our choice of foods is every bit as vital as the manner in which we consume them. Judicious food intake helps our physical condition, bolsters the body's defences against illness and also affects our mental state.

It has been calculated that, over a lifetime, the average person will ingest 30 tonnes (about 67,000 lbs) of solid food and drink roughly 50,000 litres (almost 11,000 gallons) of liquids. Clearly, the food we eat does much, much more than merely assuage our hunger or quench our thirst: our abdomen and digestive and intestinal systems continuously extract elements essential to life and protect us from infection by identifying and neutralising toxins, harmful bacteria and viruses.

We now know that our behaviour is affected and conditioned by our choice of food. We are not yet – although the day will no doubt dawn sooner or later – in a position to establish direct links between nourishment and patterns of intellectual or artistic creativity. What is beyond dispute, however, is the two-way process that occurs via neuro-transmitters. It follows that improving the performance of the abdomen will often be conducive to the alleviation of all manner of disorders and illnesses – even the most serious. Equally – and I have observed this at first hand on countless occasions – successfully treating a mental condition such as stress or anxiety will often result in better eating habits and enhanced breathing patterns, leading inevitably to a substantially healthier abdomen and digestive system.

I distinctly recall the case of a prominent chief executive who kept putting on weight, despite recourse to all manner of diets and periods of abstinence. The man was continually under pressure and incapable of relaxing. As a result, his entire digestive system had been severely disrupted. I had little difficulty in persuading him that his particular abdominal problems could be traced to his upper brain. He practised my breathing exercises on an hourly basis and, at my insistence, started to eat regularly and slowly, varying his food intake as best he could (given the constraints of obligatory business lunches and dinners). He started to eat more sensibly and followed a series of simple exercise routines I prescribed (see 'Exercises for the Two Brains' on pages 108–19). I massaged his abdomen on a regular basis and gradually succeeded

...successfully treating a mental condition such as stress or anxiety will often result in better eating habits and enhanced breathing patterns, leading inevitably to a healthier abdomen...

in bringing the two brains together. Once that happened, the extra weight quickly dropped off – for good.

Another case among the hundreds I have dealt with over the years was that of a young girl who slipped from one bout of depression into the next. She suffered from anxiety attacks and migraines and was borderline anorexic. As a photographer's model, she was in the habit of eating next to nothing and, predictably, tended to eat at irregular intervals, snatching a bite here and there whenever she had a moment during her working day. Her breathing was erratic. She also ingested various stimulants. I was not surprised to find her stomach tight and bloated. My initial priority was to massage it back into a supple, non-distended

PART II: THE METHOD

state. At the same time, I worked on her eating habits. Within a very short time, her bouts of depression became progressively less frequent, then disappeared. Her disposition changed dramatically: she became happy-go-lucky and confident, and went on to forge a splendid career for herself.

Another recent and typical case involved Jeanne, a 64-year-old businesswoman with no immediate history of personal problems. She complained of chronic lumbago and painful joints, and x-rays revealed significant arthritis in her vertebrae, hands and feet. She had already consulted a number of rheumatologists who had prescribed anti-inflammatory medication and massage therapy. Those treatments had failed and she turned to me. I quickly identified excessive cellulite (inflammation of subcutaneous tissue). She was approximately 12 kilos (26 lbs) overweight. When I palpated her abdomen, I found it hard, distended and painfully cramped. I queried Jeanne's eating habits and discovered that, over the years, she had lapsed into what I can only describe as 'anarchy'. In the morning, she drank an inordinate quantity of coffee and a large glass of fruit juice, ate white bread and jam, often with a croissant and/or brioche for good measure. Mid-morning and mid-afternoon 'treats' typically involved more coffee and biscuits. For lunch, Jeanne favoured cold cuts, fried foods and sugared desserts; dinner would include soup and a main course of meat, fish or eggs, again followed by a sugar-based pudding. She took next to no physical exercise.

I explained to Jeanne that she would have to mend her ways if she was to get back into some semblance of shape. She turned a deaf ear. 'I'm useless without my coffee,' she insisted. After three weekly sessions, I could detect no improvement whatsoever in the condition of her abdomen and I again informed her that she had to pull herself together and start eating sensibly: 'Failing that, it's pointless to continue therapy,' I said. 'A waste of time and money.' Jeanne shrugged her shoulders and left, clearly disappointed. It was a full four months before she turned up on my doorstep again. She had seen a number of other specialists, she informed me, but her condition had not improved. If anything, she was even more tired than before. This time around, she decided to take my advice. First off, no coffee. Then: eat at regular intervals and eat slowly. I advised her to eat fish, white meat, vegetables, rice, pasta and fresh fruit.

...five abdominal massage sessions later, her back pain had disappeared, her joints no longer ached, her bowel movements had regularised, she was sleeping better, and she had shed 6 kilos (13 lbs).

A month and a half and five abdominal massage sessions later, her back pain had disappeared, her joints no longer ached, her bowel movements had regularised, she was sleeping better, and she had shed 6 kilos (13 lbs). I advised her to continue following my methods, to practise my breathe-to-relax exercises, to walk one hour every day and to spend a few minutes each day massaging her abdomen. Two months later, Jeanne announced that she had lost a further 6 kilos (13 lbs). She felt in tip-top form and said as much: 'I feel great. Your approach has worked wonders so far. But for how long?' In reply, I could only suggest she adopt my two-brain exercises – with excellent results, I might add.

PART II: THE METHOD

I have direct personal experience of many cases involving eczema and psoriasis, which cleared up after milk-based products and stimulants were excluded.[16] Ear, nose and throat infections in young children can be relieved by the simple expedient of excluding sweets and sugary drinks. At the time, I may have known precious little about neuro-transmitters and the infinitesimal dosages they secrete to regulate the body, but what I did intuitively know was that co-ordinating and harmonising the two brains was frequently the path towards better health. What I also knew even back then was that better health was to a large degree dependent on being very careful in choosing what we eat and drink.

Dieting: a Word of Warning

I've spoken throughout this book about harmonising the two brains in order to promote healthy living. In practice, however, it is not as simple as it sounds. I know, because I have spent years perfecting my programme.

Point one is unequivocal: forget dieting! I am utterly opposed to any diet based on eliminating essential 'nutrients', by which I mean the fats, carbohydrates and proteins that are indispensable to the metabolic process. When, for example, I advise against dairy products, it's only for a limited period then the offending product is gradually reintroduced in homeopathic (tiny) dosages once the complaint has been successfully addressed.

It seems that everyone in the world has tried or at least heard of no-fat, no-protein, sugar-free diets, or embarked on a diet regime based exclusively on a particular product or products (such as meat or pasta, for example). This is utter madness. Any food, even food that is alleged to be 'bad' for you, has its place *somewhere.*[17]

There is sound evidence, for example, that fats – which certain diets advise you to cut out – play a major part in your sex life. There is sound evidence that carbohydrates (bread, pasta, rice, starch) have a soothing effect on the nervous system, are essential for alertness and also play a role in sexual gratification. There is sound evidence also that proteins (meat, fish, dairy products) stimulate the suprarenal glands (above the kidneys) and act directly on the upper brain to promote a feeling of well-being. And fibre – once regarded as inconsequential – is now acknowledged to be indispensable in moving nutrients along through the digestive process. Comparatively recently, it has also been demonstrated that wine (in moderate quantities) is 'good for the heart'[18].

Paracelsus, the pre-eminent man of medicine, pointed out 500 years ago that 'nothing is poison and all is poison', going on to stress that 'poison' is merely a matter of dosage. That was the beginning of homeopathy as we know it today – and we owe Paracelsus a great debt in that respect.

It may not be common knowledge, but a diet based exclusively on vegetables and fruit can be fatal if taken to extremes. Yet I have encountered young models who swear by it. Of late, reliable studies have demonstrated convincingly that suppressing one food type is enough to modify immune cell production in the abdomen, opening the door to all manner of infection. In a nutshell, eating for abdominal health is governed by three complementary considerations: food must have taste (and one that suits our personal inclinations), *variety* and *nutritional energy-building properties.*

Fibre-Rich Foods

Some fibre-rich foods remain undigested in the lower intestine. They can be classed as *soluble* (fruits and vegetables) or *insoluble* (cereal products). They slow down the digestive process because they take longer than other foods to transit the lower intestine. The fibres retain water, resulting in softer stools. They are conducive to the growth of intestinal flora and play an important part in alleviating constipation.

The utility of fibre-rich foods is uncontested. They:
- retard hunger pangs by retaining glucose, thus preventing rapid rises in blood sugar (at the same time affording increased protection against diabetes)
- effectively reduce overall food intake by around 5–10 per cent (useful when you're trying to lose weight), because they make you feel fuller
- can help to inhibit cholesterol build-up if 20 to 30 grams are eaten per day
- promote the growth and action of beneficial intestinal bacteria and counteract the production of unwanted toxins; and
- absorb or dilute carcinogenic free radicals and reduce their effect on the mucous membrane lining the intestine.

As a rule of thumb, eating more fibre-rich nutrients means increasing your intake of fruit and vegetables – gradually, so as to prevent the build-up of stomach gases – and drinking lots of mineral water to hydrate the stools (a minimum of 1.5 litres/2½ pints daily).

Carbohydrates

These are classified with reference to their effects on blood sugar levels (glycaemia) and are awarded a score in the Glycaemic Index (GI). Foods that score above 70 cause a major rise in blood sugar absorption; with those between 55 and 70, the rise is moderate; below 55, it is weak. *Simple carbohydrates* are fast-acting: sugar, jams, honey, sweetmeats, cakes, pastries, syrups, fruit, sugary drinks, juices, compotes, dairy products. Slow-acting *complex carbohydrates* include cereals: corn, wheat, barley, buckwheat, rye, rice, raw or cooked, in gruel or porridge form, or ground as flour for baking bread or pasta; vegetables and pulses: potatoes, green peas, lentils, fava beans, runner beans, soya beans, onions, garlic, salad greens, courgettes, celery, carrots; and *aromatic* herbs, such as parsley and chives.

Carbohydrates containing fibre and fats may have a lower GI score.

Most adults don't eat enough complex carbohydrates. The GI index should be used as a guide to the most nutritionally sound options.

Note: Together, simple and complex carbohydrates should represent 55 per cent of our daily food intake.

Proteins

Proteins can be animal or vegetable in origin:

Animal Protein

• Eight essential amino acids are found in both beef and lamb; the leaner cuts are recommended, since these have a lower fat content

• Poultry: free-range chicken, guinea fowl, duck, turkey
• Saltwater fish: hake, sole, cod, skate, whiting
• Freshwater fish: carp, trout, pike

Note: The fattiest kinds of fish have as high a fat content as the leanest cuts of meat.

• Crustaceans: crab, shrimp, crayfish, lobster
• Molluscs: oysters, mussels, shellfish
• Dairy products: milk, yoghurt, cheese

Vegetable Protein

• Pulses: lentils, beans, chickpeas
• Cereals: rice, corn, wholemeal pasta, wholemeal bread
• Potatoes

Note: Proteins should represent 15 per cent of our daily food intake.

Fats

These can be animal or vegetable in origin.

Saturated

• Some margarines
• Cold cuts: pâté, luncheon meats, sausages
• Fatty meat: the highest fat content is found in animals deprived of natural movement.

Unsaturated

• Margarines enriched with an 8 per cent phytosterol content can cause a 10 per cent reduction in LDL ('bad') cholesterol
• Vegetable oils: olive oil, sunflower oil, corn oil, rapeseed oil

Note: Fats should not exceed 33 per cent of our daily food intake and should preferably be of the unsaturated fatty acid variety; saturated fats should not be more than 10 per cent of our intake.

A Question of Taste

Taste is important in establishing the balance between the two brains. Professor Gershon, author of *The Second Brain*, draws attention to a neuro-transmitter that is responsible for the dual sensation of attraction and rejection. This neuro-transmitter, dopamine – discovered several years ago at Cambridge University – effectively 'regulates' taste causing us to exhibit a predilection for some foods and an aversion to others.

In a parallel development, it has also been demonstrated that, irrespective of their cultural background, newborn babies 'accept' sugar and 'reject' anything bitter. This is a curious phenomenon, all the more so since we know that in medieval times the dominant taste sensation was acidic; during the Renaissance, if leading authorities are to be believed, there was very little demand for sweet foods, and it was not until the 17th century, when the sequence of dishes during a meal was introduced, that any real distinction was made between sweet and savoury dishes. The major – and catastrophic – trend towards excessive sugar consumption dates from the 1950s, just after World War II.

It has also been established that the foetus develops taste organs during the fourth month in the womb. Boris Cyrulnik, the celebrated behavioural scientist and psychiatrist from Marseilles University, has proved that newborn infants from that city respond positively to a nipple tasting of garlic if it is eaten by the mother during pregnancy, but this phenomenon is not shown by newborns in Paris, where the mothers did not eat garlic during pregnancy. It follows that it is important to educate the tastebuds of young children as early as possible.[19]

At one point it was thought that children could eat virtually anything, provided that they developed normally. Infants have in excess of 10,000 taste cells, around half of which will be lost before they reach adulthood. It is important to experience a broad range of tastes during infancy if the subsequent adult tastebuds are to be properly educated.[20]

Parents who indulge childhood preferences for sweet foods often cause dramatic consequences in later life. This is particularly true in the United States, the home of fast food, where parents frequently allow their children convenience foods such as tomato ketchup, sugary sweets and fizzy drinks. In Europe also, the number of overweight and obese children has doubled over the past decade and continues to increase.

Adult abdominal health is conditioned by childhood eating habits. In adults, excess body weight significantly increases the risk of diabetes and heart disease. Quite recently, research at INSERM, the Paris-based institute for the study of diabetes, has identified the benefits of 'preventative nutrition', a concept of which I wholeheartedly approve. It is now accepted that carefully selected and well-balanced nutrition stimulates two-brain harmony and reduces the incidence of a number of illnesses, particularly cardiovascular disorders, cancers and osteoporosis. Professor Serge Reynauld has demonstrated that a diet that is low in saturated fats but enriched by polyunsaturated linoleic acids (the 'Cretan' diet) affords a high level of protection.[21] Choosing fresh natural foods, such as avocados, nuts, seeds and oily fish will provide these 'good' fats.

My first rule regarding the choice of food is to let your taste-buds dictate what you eat. In other words, go for what you genuinely like, giving free rein to the senses, but always in moderation. This will ensure that your upper and lower brains are in tune. It is now accepted that what we call 'appetite' is directly stimulated by the two brains working in tandem via several neuro-transmitters, and that specific 'cravings' – for sugar, salt, fruit, chocolate, meat and so on – are, in virtually every case, no more than the body's need for a specific nutrient. In a nutshell, we eat what we want and need. This is yet another example of the balance between the upper and lower brains.

...stimulants such as tobacco or alcohol... disrupt the body's natural nutritional needs, destroy vitamins, and frequently cause serious dysfunctions and excess weight gain or loss.

However, stimulants such as tobacco or alcohol upset this precarious balance, disrupt the body's natural nutritional needs, destroy vitamins, and frequently cause serious dysfunctions and excess weight gain or loss. It is for this reason that tobacco should be avoided and alcohol intake restricted to wine consumed in moderation during a meal.

Excess and the Abdomen

The Paris-based INSERM research unit has recently released findings about the effects of alcohol, coffee, tea and tobacco on various metabolic processes.[22] The conclusions are fascinating, not least because of the complex relationship identified in each case

PART II: THE METHOD

between the abdomen and the upper brain. Closer study of the neuro-transmitters involved shows clearly that this relationship is a two-way street. For example, alcohol works on the abdomen via the upper brain and vice-versa. Specialists have discovered that problems arising from excess alcohol consumption are 'circulated' in parallel via the neuro-transmitters in the two brains and that the impact of such excessive consumption is equally divided between them.[23]

Logically, the same holds true when our body takes in excessive amounts of sugar or other products such as coffee or tea, or ingests carcinogenic tobacco smoke. In each instance, research points to the benefits of avoiding excess. INSERM's findings reconfirm the importance of a balanced interdependency between the two brains and, in consequence, the importance that must always attach to conditioning the abdomen.

A Varied, Energy-Rich and High Nutrient Value Diet

Our eating habits may be dictated by taste but we need a range of foods that are fresh, healthy, and with optimal vitamin, mineral and trace element content. I have never advised cutting out any specific food, although I have stipulated that tea, coffee, honey and jams should be taken in moderation. Where certain dysfunctions or illnesses are concerned (see Part III), I advise abstention from some foods until the abdomen returns to health. A healthy abdomen absorbs and eliminates every type of food and its intestinal flora will reconstitute to combat any hostile bacteria. It can also deal with excessive intake of alcoholic beverages or tobacco-related stimulants – provided such excessive intake does not become habitual. Indulging from time to time is not a danger and I even believe that the resulting enjoyment is conducive to two-brain equilibrium.

It is important to pay attention to food hygiene, because food can be altered or contaminated by pathogens, bacteria, mould and other toxins. Fruit and vegetables should be washed to get rid of pesticide residues on the skin. Be wary of genetically modified foodstuffs and keep your consumption of them to a minimum.

Much depends on how each food is prepared and cooked. Protracted cooking times destroy vitamins and reduce energy-generating qualities. Barbecues, which produce charred meats, fish and potatoes, should be avoided. Charred foods are a source of free radicals (see below), which kill cells, accelerate the age-ing process and can cause cancer. Cooking oils should be clear and filtered before re-use (and should not be re-used more than once or twice). Cooking with fats, such as butter and lard, should be avoided as they destabilise the digestive tracts and bile ducts. Fruits and vegetables that are peeled, grated or sliced should be eaten within a quarter of an hour, or the vitamin content will degrade in a process of oxidation (see below).

Free Radicals versus Antioxidants

The role played by 'free radicals' in cell mutation was identified some 40 years ago. Since then, researchers have assigned them progressively greater responsibility in this respect.

Free radicals oxidise – as it were 'rust' – all our cells. Atoms are the building block of molecules, which in turn are the building blocks of cells. Normal atoms consist of a nucleus, neutrons, (positively charged) protons and (negatively charged) electrons. In molecules, certain electrons tend to be paired but, in the

PART II: THE METHOD

case of free radicals, they work unpaired. As a result, there are unattached electrons. These are highly unstable and react with other compounds, searching out a 'mate'. In the process, they attack and destroy the nearest stable molecule. This is known as oxidation.

Free radicals are at the root of numerous illnesses. Although they have a very short lifespan – often less than a second – they are highly dangerous. According to the Kings College biochemist Barry Halliwell, the human body produces some 2 kilograms (4 lbs) of free radicals annually, with an estimated 5 per cent of oxygen intake transformed into free radicals. We absorb still more through polluted atmospheres, harmful radiation from the sun, exposure to pollutants, and ingested or inhaled toxins – typically from inadequately preserved, oxidised or processed food, tobacco and so on.

Each of our body's cells is attacked several hundred times a day. Fortunately, the body has defence mechanisms to ward off such attacks: antioxidants. The major antioxidants are vitamins A (beta-carotene), C and E, together with the minerals selenium, iron and zinc, and other substances such as polyphenols, flavonoids, carotenoids, anthocyanins and tannins. These substances are present in our cells, where their role is to prevent or repair damage caused by free radicals. Careful nutritional choices can ensure we have plenty of these antioxidants.

Recent research has shown that our defence system is designed to maintain a continual level of protection against free radicals. Sadly, that is not always the case in practice. Under conditions of stress or fatigue, overwork, ageing, menopause, insufficient nutrition and poor breathing techniques – in other words, when the two brains are out of synch – free radicals have a field day. The immune system can weaken, opening the door to illness and accelerated ageing. Antioxidants play a key role in the body's defence against cardiovascular, microbial or cancerous conditions and against the ageing process.

INSERM research[24] clearly demonstrates the importance of eating fruit and vegetables as a key source of antioxidants. However, antioxidants taken in the form of mega-vitamins or other supplements deliver substantially higher doses than those derived from natural foodstuffs and can actually prove harmful to health.[25]

It is best to get adequate vitamins naturally, from your food.

Free radicals are at the root of numerous illnesses. Although they have a very short lifespan – often less than a second – they are highly dangerous.

See the information on vitamins that follows to ensure you are consuming foods from each category.

Antioxidant Vitamins

Vitamin A

This vitamin combats oxidation, ageing and infection. It helps to renew the skin, hair and nails and is vital for healthy bones, teeth and gums. It protects the membrane walls of the digestive and respiratory tracts and appears to reduce the risk of cardiovascular malfunction.

The body coverts carotene (the pigment present in fruit and green, yellow and red vegetables) into provitamin A or beta-

carotene. Carotene is present in:
- *green vegetables*: spinach, French beans, broccoli, peas, cabbage, salad leaves
- *aromatic herbs*: parsley, coriander, chives, basil, chervil
- *yellow or red vegetables*: peppers, carrots, squash, tomatoes, onions, shallots, garlic
- *fruits*: peaches, mangoes, apricots, melons, bananas.

Vitamins B_1, B_5, B_6

These protect the skin and are used by the nervous system to ward off stress, depression, insomnia and anxiety. These vitamins help to convert carbohydrates and fats into energy. They need vitamin C to be effective, and they interact positively with magnesium. They are present in:
- raw vegetables, cereals, yeast, wheatgerm.

Vitamin C

This stimulates cell regeneration and is important for skin, bones and teeth. It is anti-bacterial and anti-viral, reinforces the immune system and promotes longevity. Vitamin C is a major antioxidant, which counters chain reactions triggered by free radicals. Vitamin C efficacy is heightened by the presence of vitamin E and beta-carotene. It is present in:
- *fruits:* oranges, lemons, grapefruit, bananas, grapes, strawberries, raspberries, gooseberries, cherries, blackcurrants, blueberries, apples, pears
- *vegetables*: radishes, carrots, broccoli, cress, cabbage, peppers, all greens
- *aromatic herbs.*

Vitamin E

Essential for the development and protection of cell membranes. Prevents ageing and protects against cardiovascular problems. Reinforces the immune system. Compatible with vitamin C and prolongs the effects of vitamin A (beta-carotene). It is found in:
• olive oil, sunflower oil, wheatgerm, peanut oil, soya
• vegetables and fruits
• walnuts, hazelnuts, almonds, peanuts.

Antioxidant Trace Elements

These combat ageing and reinforce the cardiovascular and immune systems. They include:

Selenium

It needs vitamins A, C and E to be effective. It is present in:
• *cereals*: wheatgerm, yeast
• *vegetables*: broccoli, garlic, onion, cabbage
• *nuts*: walnuts, hazelnuts, almonds

Zinc

Essential for the production of certain enzymes. Acts on the digestive metabolism. Affects moods and stimulates the sex glands. Accelerates formation of scar tissue and helps combat teenage acne. Complements and intensifies the action of vitamins A and B. It is present in:
• *vegetables*: French beans, peas, cabbage, cress, broccoli, spinach, carrots, beetroot, onions, shallots, garlic
• wholemeal cereals, wholemeal bread, lentils
• fish, seafood, meat, poultry.

A Word of Caution

Antioxidants are sensitive to light, heat and humidity. They are destroyed if food is cooked for a long period or with an excessive amount of water. When a fruit or vegetable is peeled or juiced, it oxidises in a matter of ten minutes. Antioxidants are also destroyed by alcohol and tobacco.

Three Breakfast Menus for Two-Brain Harmony

Together with my wife Florence, I have compiled three 'abdomen-friendly' breakfast menus to kick-start the day:

- *an antacid breakfast to detox the system*
- *a light breakfast to reinvigorate the system; and*
- *an energy-rich breakfast to boost the system.*

Feel free to opt for any of them depending on your current state of health, energy levels, and overall mental or physical condition. The menus are detailed on pages 92–7.

An Antacid Breakfast to Detox the System

To be eaten while sitting down in restful surroundings; always eat the solids first.

One boiled free-range egg
or *one slice of ham*
or *one slice of chicken*
or *one portion of hard cheese*
or *one portion of goat's cheese*
or *one natural yoghurt*

One or two slices of wholemeal, granary, rye or non-wheat bread
or *one bowl of plain rice*
or *one portion of pasta*

Fresh butter
Fresh herbs (chives, parsley, basil, coriander)
One alkaline seasonal fruit (apple, banana, peach)
2 or 3 dates **or** *figs* **or** *raisins* **or** *almonds* **or** *grapes* **or** *plums*

An infusion of thyme, rosemary and sage
or *an infusion* **or** *verbena* **or** *lime-blossom* **or** *chicory*

NOTE: Until your system stabilises, you must avoid the following:

• sugar-based products: honey, jams, chocolate spread
• pastries, croissants, muffins, cakes, biscuits
• white bread
• all varieties of toasted bread (the carbonisation makes this less healthy)
• all breakfast cereals
• dairy products: milk, cream, pasteurised cheese, fruit yoghurts
• stimulants: coffee, tea, drinking chocolate
• mint tea
• fruit juices (even freshly squeezed); these don't give the saliva time to work on them in the stomach
• pre-prepared fruit salads
• fried foods, including chips; and
• delicatessen products such as pâtés, sausages or bacon.

This breakfast menu is conducive to a healthier abdomen and will help to combat joint and ligament inflammation, tendinitis, neuritis and back pain. It can also ease arthritis, and certain nervous complaints, such as irritability and anxiety.

The antacid breakfast routine should be followed until symptoms have completely disappeared. It can be followed for several weeks or months, or even permanently if you suffer from a chronic illness.

PART II: THE METHOD

A Light Breakfast to Reinvigorate the System

To be eaten while sitting down in restful surroundings; always eat the solids first.

One boiled free-range egg
or *one portion of goat's cheese*
or *one portion of cream cheese*
or *one natural yoghurt*

One or two slices of wholemeal, granary or non-wheat bread
Fresh butter

Fresh herbs (chives, parsley, basil, coriander)
One fresh seasonal fruit (orange, grapefruit, apple, peeled peach, mango or kiwi)
or *one glass of squeezed fruit juice with pulp, (try*
$1/3$ orange, $1/3$ grapefruit, $1/3$ lemon)

One tea or coffee (add milk only if you can tolerate it)
or *one herbal infusion*
or *chicory*

NOTE: Until your system stabilises, you must avoid the following:

- sugar-based products: honey, jams, chocolate spread, sweets
- pastries, croissants, muffins, cakes, biscuits
- white bread
- dairy products: milk, chocolate milk, fruit yoghurts or natural yoghurt sweetened with honey, jam, fruit or chocolate
- canned fruit juices or juices with sugar substitutes
- fried foods, including chips
- sauces
- melted cheese dishes, such as fondue
- delicatessen products such as pâté and sausages.

This light breakfast menu promotes abdominal health, rests the digestive system and will help you to lose weight, eliminate fatigue, combat diabetes, lower bad cholesterol levels and prevent cardiovascular disorders. The regime should be followed for several weeks or even months until your ideal weight is restored and your overall feeling of well-being reinstated. The menu is good for those who have been eating or drinking excessively and is ideally suited to those who prefer not to eat too much first thing in the morning.

PART II: THE METHOD

An Energy-Rich Breakfast to Boost the System

To be eaten while sitting down in restful surroundings; always eat the solids first.

One or two free-range boiled eggs
or *one omelette* fines herbes
or *one serving of fried eggs and bacon*
or *one portion of chicken breast*
or *one slice of ham (on the bone)*
or *one portion of cheese*
or *one fish fillet (salmon, herring)*

One dairy product – either milk, cream cheese or yoghurt

Two or three slices of wholemeal or granary bread
or *one bowl of rice or plate of pasta*
or *a bowl of cereal (such as cornflakes)*
Fresh butter
Fresh aromatic herbs (chives, parsley, basil, coriander)

One fresh seasonal fruit (banana, apple, pear, peach, grapefruit, orange, mango, kiwi)
or *one glass of freshly squeezed fruit with pulp*
or *2 or 3 dates, figs, almonds, walnuts, hazelnuts or prunes*

Honey or home-made low-sugar jam
Tea or coffee (with or without milk)
Chicory **or** *a herbal infusion*

NOTE: Until your system stabilises, you must avoid the following:

• pastries and biscuits
• white bread
• dried fruits or nuts with added salt, honey or caramel (dried apricots are particularly difficult to digest); and
• pre-prepared fruit salads.

This energy-intensive breakfast menu is good for boosting the immune defences by providing a large intake of vitamins, trace elements and minerals. It is designed to build overall fitness and combat stress, fatigue, depression, nervous disorders and anxiety. It can also be used to regain weight after an illness or an operation. It is recommended before sustained physical or intellectual exercise and has a calmative effect on the central nervous system. It is particularly good for harmonising the two brains. This breakfast menu should only be selected when illnesses or disorders have been addressed and abdominal health restored via the 'antacid' and 'light' breakfast menus. Don't follow it for more than two or three weeks at a time.

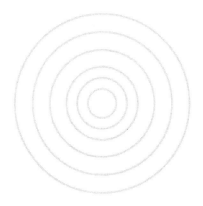

RECREATIONAL EXERCISE

A WELL-KNOWN ACTOR, who would no doubt prefer to remain anonymous, once came to consult me. He was talented, popular and had a great career ahead of him, but he was suffering from headaches and stomach pains and felt completely run-down, unable to get a decent night's sleep and wake up refreshed. His doctor had examined him at length and had pronounced him – to his consternation – 'in excellent form'. When he turned up on my doorstep, he was obviously worried about his general health which, he asserted, seemed to be of little concern to anyone else – not even to his wife, herself a famous actress.

It didn't take me long to get to the bottom of things. The man was paying the price of celebrity, footing the bill for a life lived in overdrive. At the time, he was acting in a play between two film shoots. He ate on a hit-or-miss basis, chain-smoked, drank to excess and had regular recourse to stimulants. It was pointless suggesting to him that he change the habits of a lifetime – for him, that would have required a complete personality change. His abdomen was rigid and distended and it was immediately apparent that his lower and upper brains were out of synch.

I started him on a course of intense abdominal massage and he seemed to be pleased with the results, confiding to me after a few sessions that, if nothing else, he was sleeping better. The notion of a connection between his two brains seemed to mystify him, however. I managed to persuade him to practise my breathe-to-relax exercises, stage and film work permitting. As a professional actor, abdominal breathing was a concept he could readily relate to. I also suggested he took some light exercise each morning and I explained that he would have to take up some sort of recreational exercise and practise it once a week.

Like so many of my patients in his age bracket (between forty and sixty years), he had participated in a variety of sports in his younger days, including cycling, swimming and amateur soccer. He had progressively abandoned these pursuits as the day-to-day pressures of his professional life intensified and as he became increasingly successful. He agreed to take up cycling each Sunday, however, and he also spent an hour or two walking in the woods with his wife. After a few weeks, he announced that he was feeling better.

'I know,' I replied. 'I can tell by your abdomen.'

Ever since then, a Sunday morning bicycle ride has become an essential part of his routine. Even when he is on location, he makes arrangements to cycle at least once a week. His wife (whom I also treated) told me she had decided to follow suit and that, since then, her digestion had improved. On top of that, she was sleeping more soundly than before. 'As far as I can tell,' she said one day, 'it seems that exercising my legs and breathing better have freed up my head!'

I can think of no better illustration of the link between our two brains. Moderate exercise involving an endurance sport stimulates the interaction between the two brains via the vagus nerve and benefits the entire body.

In this context, 'endurance sport' is taken to mean a sport or other activity that is practised consistently but in moderation, so that the heart rate is raised for a minimum of 45 minutes, *without* any sudden spurts or decelerations.

Moderate exercise involving an endurance sport stimulates the interaction between the two brains via the vagus nerve and benefits the entire body.

I can scarcely remember all the cases I have witnessed where very serious functional disorders (persistent fatigue, back pain, insomnia, sexual dysfunction and the like) have simply vanished by the simple expedient of exercising regularly. Recreational exercise boosts the intake of oxygen to the bloodstream and builds resistance to toxins. Both the respiratory system and the cardiovascular system are fortified. You sleep better. Muscles are toned. I have seen patients look younger, slim down, and regain a fresher and healthier skin tone. In younger patients, I have seen chronic acne and allergies disappear. At the same time, they all feel better, thanks to the beneficial effects on the upper brain. Anxieties ebb away, self-awareness and self-confidence are restored and, in very many instances, all traces of being 'run down' promptly disappear.

The worried parents of an 18-year-old student approached me one day, explaining that their son, a very bright young man, habitually spent six to eight hours a day at his computer. He was overweight, unable to shed the excess weight and had great difficulty sleeping without recourse to medication. While working on his abdomen, I asked a few pertinent questions. It emerged he had once been a passionate devotee of roller blading, but that he had given up two years previously because he had 'too many other things on his plate'. I advised him to take up roller blading again and to practise his favourite sport at least three times a week. He took my advice and over the next few months he lost 6 kilos (13 lbs) and could sleep soundly without popping sleeping pills. In essence, he had 're-aligned' his two brains.

When all is said and done, however, it is at the level of the abdomen that the effects are most rapid and direct. There is no abdominal malfunction (constipation, wind, severe menstrual cramps and so on) that will not respond positively to regular and moderate recreational exercise. Taken in conjunction with the other essential elements of my method – breathing, proper nutrition, and so forth – the improvement will be even more spectacular.

A Closer Look at Endurance Sports

Physical activity in the form of an endurance sport generates the production of endorphins ('feel-good' hormones), stabilises blood pressure, strengthens the cardiovascular and respiratory systems, relaxes the central nervous system (the upper brain) and combats certain undesirable psychological states, including anxiety, shyness and fear of failure. The benefits of endurance sport have been convincingly demonstrated in the battle against diabetes, undesirable weight gain and the reduction of 'bad' cholesterol. Additionally, practising an endurance sport boosts the immune system.

Before each session, you should 'warm up' with five to six minutes of gentle stretching exercises. These should be repeated at the end of each session to avoid stresses and strains and the accumulation of excess acid in the muscles and joints. Working out on a regular basis for, say, a 45-minute period should not make you tired or out of breath. Each session can be punctuated by an *occasional* burst of acceleration: for example, gentle and sustained exercise for 20 minutes or so may be followed by a two-to-three-minute sprint before returning to the earlier pace. This may be repeated two to three times during a 45-minute workout, while the heart rate is monitored. Working out in this way effectively doubles the benefits to the body as a whole.

Walking, cycling and swimming are all very beneficial, but excessive jogging and 'extreme' sports can damage the muscles and joints, place undue strain on the heart or provoke abdominal malfunction. Never go beyond your limits, or start exercising without a warm-up. More often than not, jogging exacerbates pre-existing complaints, intensifying fatigue and making you look older. I'm not saying, 'Don't jog at all', but it is essential that you are in good shape before you take up a jogging programme, that you warm up properly and don't over-exert yourself.

A healthy abdomen and a well-regulated heartbeat (see the section on self-massage on page 120) are essential before you take up running, and it's important to build up your speed and distance gradually. The same holds true for swimming and, to an extent, tennis. In stop-start games like tennis, it is important to choose a pace and intensity that don't over-exert you. You can decide whether to chase a ball or not, depending on your heart rate and how your abdomen is feeling. If the abdomen is in poor shape, the link to the upper brain will be broken and the system will malfunction. This happens even at the top levels of sport, causing 'super-fit' athletes to collapse suddenly within yards of the finishing line. Their reserves of abdominal energy have become exhausted, causing the upper brain to disconnect. Some turn to artificial and illegal substances to try to prevent this, a practice I find regrettable.

Athletes and the Upper Brain

Many athletes, even those at the pinnacle of their sport, pay too little attention to their abdomen. They are ill-advised, as building abdominal health into their training regime should be a prime consideration in order to improve performance, prevent muscle strains, eliminate lapses in concentration and prolong their athletic career.

Leading athletes are often prone to nutritional errors and misconceptions. They should not eat as much when they are not in training and competition or they will put on unwanted weight; if they eat too sparingly they increase the risk of muscle strain because they will not absorb enough vitamins and energy-providing glucose; eating an excess of simple, fast-acting sugars, such as chocolate bars and sweets, fermented cheese and fried foods is harmful; insufficient liquid intake leads to dehydration; an insufficiency of proteins in the form of poultry, fish, white meat and calcium-rich milk products will make it difficult to maintain muscle strength; and eating an insufficient quantity of essential fatty acids, such as those present in olive oil, will weaken the system.

My advice to athletes is to eat four or five times a day during periods of intense training and competition and to follow a regime based on complex carbohydrates (wholegrain rice, pasta and potatoes), together with sufficient fruits and vegetables to provide the essential antioxidants (see pages 85–90).

Selecting a Recreational Sport

Choose any endurance sport that you enjoy. If practised prudently and in moderation, it will be conducive to abdominal health. This is in part because sporting activity gives a natural massage, which

> **I favour exercising outdoors to engage all the senses. At all costs, avoid cluttered, airless, noisy surroundings... find a green space that is calm, secure and quiet.**

helps stimulate abdominal functions and, as a result, induces proper interaction between the two brains.

Practise your chosen sport in agreeable surroundings. Personally, I favour exercising outdoors to engage all the senses. At all costs, avoid cluttered, airless, noisy surroundings. I attach major importance to environment, since this is vital to stimulate the upper brain. Even if you live in a city, it is usually possible to find a green space nearby that is calm, secure and, with any luck, quiet.

A study published in 2001 by Duke University, North Carolina[26], followed 30 subjects under the age of 30 who were all taking antidepressants. Half were encouraged to embark instead on an undemanding sports programme involving 20-minute gym sessions and regular short outings on foot or by bicycle. The conclusions of the study showed that those following the exercise option exhibited identical positive reactions to those still on anti-depressants. It is clear to me that the two brains were 'desynchronised' and had then been brought back together again through exercise.

Recreational Sport: the Ten Commandments

1. If you are not the sporting type or if you have not indulged in sport for over a year, start with short sessions of activity (ten to fifteen minutes at a time). Stop at the first sign of tiredness, pain or breathing difficulties.

2. Whatever sport you choose, start off by 'unclogging' with the Two-Brain Exercises (see pages 114–9) in order to stimulate the liver and bile ducts. This will help to prevent stitches, a sign that your digestive system is not in tune with the activity in question. If you do get a stitch, simply walk gently and breathe deeply. If the stitch persists, stop what you are doing and try again the following day.

3. After the first two or three weeks, you may safely increase the length of sessions. You will quickly move to 45 minutes and beyond. I recommend a minimum of 45 minutes since this is the time required to free up the endorphins that are indispensable to restoring or sustaining two-brain harmony.

4. Never exercise to excess. You are not in a competitive situation; instead, your goal is merely to enjoy yourself and promote your own well-being.

5. Never allow your heart to race and never exercise to the point where you feel abdominal pain. To check your pulse, press your fingers (not your thumb) lightly on the vein in your opposite

PART II: THE METHOD

wrist just below the thumb. You should feel it pulsate. Count the number of beats in fifteen seconds, then multiply by four to determine the number of beats per minute. The normal pulse rate at rest is between 66 and 75 beats/minute for a man and between 75 and 83 for a woman. During physical exertion, this rate should never be permitted to exceed 150 (man or woman) and, if you are over 50, keep it below 140. Once physical activity stops, the pulse rate should gradually return to normal. However, if your pulse rate does not decrease below 120 after five minutes have elapsed, this could indicate that you have exercised too long and too hard for your physical condition. Reduce the duration and intensity of the exercise next time.

6. After exercising, test your abdomen by positioning your hands on either side of the navel, inhaling gently and following my breathe-to-relax method. There should be no abdominal pain whatsoever. If you are unable to inhale for a period of seven or eight seconds or exhale for between eight and ten seconds, walk about (slowly) to recover from the excess effort expended.

7. If you start to pant, stop exercising immediately and walk about slowly, breathing in and out as described in point 6.

8. When walking or running, wear shoes with impact-absorbing soles. Don't wear too many clothes. Drink liquids before and after exercising, taking care not to gulp too quickly. Liquids shouldn't be too hot or too cold, as this causes stomach acid build-up, prompts the sphincter to open and can make you feel exhausted. Inhale every two paces and exhale over the following three. Your posture should be upright, with chest out and shoulders relaxed. Arms should move loosely in time to the pace at which you are walking or running. Note

that you should walk after a meal rather than run; walking speeds up the digestive process, whereas running inhibits it. Try to walk for at least half an hour daily.

9. When cycling, choose your bike carefully, and make sure the saddle is in the correct position so that you sit with good posture. Never cycle on an empty stomach and note that wearing a belt restricts abdominal breathing. Avoid wearing belts or restrictive clothing while exercising. If you are cycling a long distance, have something to eat and drink every 25 kilometres (15 miles). Be careful not to expose the abdomen to low temperatures; wear a wind-cheater.

10. Swimming is the sport best suited to developing and sustaining two-brain harmony. Aim to have a 20- to 30-minute swim twice a week in warm water or, better still, seawater.

You should feel the difference soon after you start following these recommendations regularly. Note that I attach particular importance to exercising for more than 45 minutes. This is the point at which you will get what athletes loosely refer to as their 'second wind', an expression which describes the pleasurable sensation on the full release of endorphins, which ensure the body's various organs, glands and systems are functioning optimally.

The first 20 minutes of exercise is about warming up the muscles, after which the upper brain gradually relaxes. The next 20 minutes stimulate bodily functions, improve the circulation and deliver the energy required to develop 'second wind'. If this plateau is not reached, the beneficial effects for the two brains will not be attained. Typically, it takes 45 minutes of exercise for the body's metabolism to peak and for the two brains to harmonise.

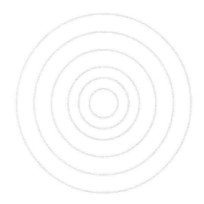

EXERCISES FOR THE TWO BRAINS

IT IS SOME YEARS NOW SINCE I FIRST formulated my psychological therapy based on isometric movements and exercises. At the time, I was unaware of the intimate interaction that medical research has since confirmed between the upper brain and our second brain, the abdomen, by way of neuro-transmitters operating via the vagus nerve.

When my intuitive approach received 'official' recognition, my reaction was twofold. First, I had the satisfaction of being able to comprehend more fully the positive results I had achieved up to that point; and, second, I was inspired to take my method a step further by integrating the abdomen into these psychological exercises. The concept I now term 'two-brain exercises' was born.

In essence, the concept is based on exercise with a spiritual dimension. Even those who hate physical exercise have found it both pleasurable and efficient.

Imagined Movements

Initially, the idea was to develop a sequence of movements based on natural movements that are used routinely in rural environments: chopping wood, drawing water from a well, binding sheaves, driving in fence-posts, pushing or pulling objects or lifting heavy loads. In times gone by, this type of physical exertion contributed to the elimination of stress and aggression, reduced tensions and helped calm the central nervous system. A sense of healthy physical tiredness induced a sense of psychological well-being.

Since we can't all step backwards and live life the way our ancestors did, I developed 'imaginary' exercises where these gestures were performed not physically but 'in the mind's eye'. As a result, you could 'exercise' anywhere – at home, in the office, in the car, on the train or when travelling by plane. All it required was that the spinal column was slightly rounded and the legs bent. This position enables the abdomen to inflate and deflate optimally.

Over the years, my psychological approach has been vindicated by the successful treatment of countless conditions ranging from back pain to abdominal complaints, insomnia to diminished libido and unwanted weight gain, nervous anxiety to low self-confidence. Once a scientific explanation of the role of the abdomen had been advanced, I developed my method, inviting patients to imagine that they were using their abdomen to move a weight up and down during the inhalation-exhalation cycle. I quickly found that this 'two-brain' approach yielded significant

PART II: THE METHOD

results, both physical and psychological:

- Gastrointestinal aches and pains, wind, cramps and constipation disappeared.
- Cellulite on the abdomen, hips, thighs and waist was eliminated.
- Unwanted body weight was shed and abdominal and overall muscle tone enhanced.
- The rectus abdominus muscle, which links the sternum and the pubic area, stimulates the digestive system and creates a flatter abdomen, was strengthened.
- There was a drop in harmful cholesterol levels, increasingly stable blood pressure, and an overall reinforcement of the cardiovascular, pulmonary and digestive systems.
- There was increased suppleness in the spinal column as inter-vertebral discs, each of which connects to a system, organ or gland, were progressively released. Spinal blockage of any sort leads to abdominal dysfunction.
- Diminished vulnerability to type 2 diabetes was noted. An article in the *New England Journal of Medicine*[27] postulated that a 30-minute walk was more efficacious than medication in the control of diabetes. Studies involving members of a Native American tribe with diabetes demonstrated that simply flexing the arm for a total of one hour daily was every bit as effective as an insulin injection.
- The hormonal and immune systems were strengthened.
- Physical abilities when playing sport were improved.
- A decrease in or elimination of nervous tension and depression was recorded.
- There was an increased response to psychotherapy; and, generally, closer harmonisation of the two brains.

Abdomen and Back

The abdomen connects directly to the spinal column; as a result, a healthy abdomen depends on a healthy back. Nerves issuing from apertures in the spinal vertebrae each correspond to a specific abdominal system, organ or gland. In the event of an aperture becoming blocked, the corresponding function will suffer. A blockage between the fourth and fifth vertebrae, for example, will affect the liver and stomach and lead to circulatory problems. When a blockage occurs, frequently as a result of compacted inter-vertebral discs, abdominal health is impaired – at which point it is time to consult an osteopath, chiropractor, physiotherapist, kinesiologist, acupuncturist or sports doctor.

One case among the hundreds I have personally dealt with over the years involved a man named Jérôme, who was 35 years old and suffering from back pain. He was fully aware that osteopathy is rooted in the principle that disorders can be alleviated by manipulation and massage of the human skeleton and musculature. What he did not seem to grasp, however, was that his problem could not be alleviated in a single session. I had to explain at length that, in order to treat his back and avoid a relapse, the first priority was to do something about his abdomen. Jérôme ate too quickly and took next to no exercise. As a result, his waistline had expanded, and the excess weight he carried around his middle was putting a strain on his lumbar vertebrae and distorting his posture. I encouraged him to practise my two-brain exercises twice daily. Several weeks and sessions later, he had exercised his abdomen back to full health. His waistline had firmed up and his stomach was flat. He had taken to eating slowly and in a relaxed state. His back pain was a thing of the past.

PART II: THE METHOD

Maintain an upright posture when repeating the following basic exercise, which can be done at virtually any time of day.

Simple Breathing Exercise for the Abdomen

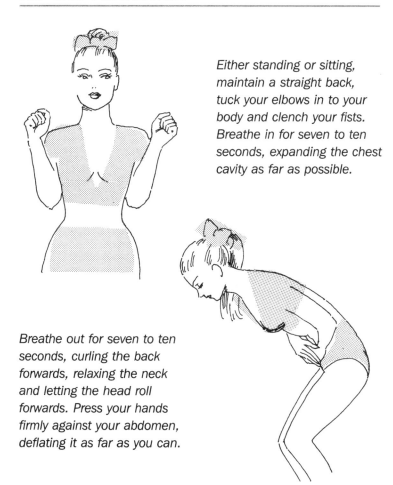

Either standing or sitting, maintain a straight back, tuck your elbows in to your body and clench your fists. Breathe in for seven to ten seconds, expanding the chest cavity as far as possible.

Breathe out for seven to ten seconds, curling the back forwards, relaxing the neck and letting the head roll forwards. Press your hands firmly against your abdomen, deflating it as far as you can.

Two-Brain Exercises

In practice, two-brain exercises can be performed in a standing, sitting or reclining position. Routines should be followed twice daily, before breakfast and prior to the evening meal. They can also be followed when you need to relax to ward off stress.

Remove your jacket, free the abdomen from any constraints and try to shut out the outside world. Note that movement should first be envisaged in the mind's eye and thought through at the level of the upper brain, before being executed by the lower brain (the abdomen). Each exercise is a continuous sequence of slow and meaningful movements synchronised with abdominal breathing patterns.

The two-brain approach advocated here initially requires a considerable level of self-control. Accordingly, I counsel a slow and measured start in the early sessions and an increase in intensity over time. The French actor Gérard Depardieu was introduced to my method during a television programme and acknowledged that he felt the benefits right there and then.

Note: When practising exercises the following scale is useful:

    ● = easy

    ●● = slightly more difficult

    ●●● = moderately difficult

    ●●●● = requires concentration/difficult

PART II: THE METHOD

Exercise 1:
Full-Body Sequence

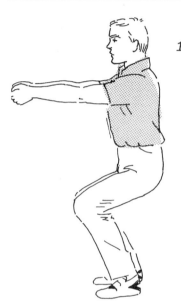

1. Stand upright with your feet hip-width apart and bend your knees, imagining your feet pressing into the ground. Clench your buttocks and rock the pelvis and pubic area forwards and upwards. The back should be slightly rounded, the arms held straight out in front and the shoulders relaxed.

2. Make a fist with each hand and imagine you are pulling something towards you (heavy or not, the upper brain will decide). At the same time, breathe in slowly through the nose for seven to ten seconds and inflate the abdomen as if you are pushing against a load.

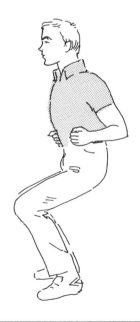

3. *After seven to ten seconds, lower the fists to waist level, tucking in the elbows; hold this position for one or two seconds.*

4. *Unclench your fists and push the imaginary load away from you, breathing out for seven to ten seconds. At the same time, curve your back forwards, let your head fall forwards between your arms, and expel as much air as possible from your abdomen, to the point where your navel seems to be pressing against your spine.*

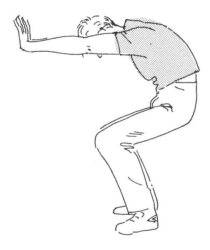

The above sequence should be repeated five times a day at first then increase to seven or eight times daily after a few days. Unless you are a trained athlete, never exceed twelve to fifteen repetitions.

Exercise 2:
Abdomen and Back

1. *Kneel on all fours on a thick carpet, with your legs slightly apart and palms pressing down into the floor. Breathe in for seven to ten seconds, inflating the abdomen, and imagine you are pushing a heavy load into the ground beneath you.*

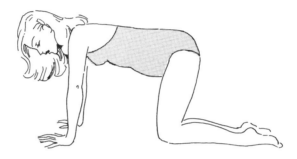

2. *Breathe out for seven to ten seconds, imagining that your abdomen is pulling the load upwards, and think about pulling your navel back towards the spinal column. Curve your back upwards and let your head drop between your outstretched arms.*

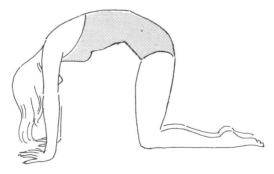

3. *Repeat five times, pause, then start again, performing the full sequence two or three times over.*

Exercise 3:
Abdominal Muscles

1. *Lie on your back on a thick carpet and bend your knees, resting your arms by your sides. Breathe in for seven to ten seconds, inflating the abdomen and imagining that you are pushing a weight upwards.*

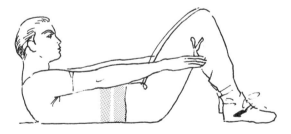

2. *Raise the upper body from the floor and stretch your arms forwards so that your hands go past your thighs. Remain in this position as you exhale for seven to ten seconds, imagining that a weight is pressing down on your abdomen.*

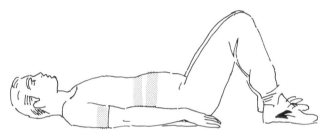

3. *Repeat five times, pause, then perform the full sequence two or three times over.*

PART II: THE METHOD

Exercise 4:
Abdomen and Waist

1. *Lie on your back, knees bent, on a thick carpet. Rest the left heel on the right knee and clasp your hands behind your neck, with your elbows wide. Breathe in for seven to ten seconds, inflating the abdomen and imagining that you are pushing a weight upwards.*

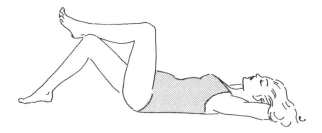

2. *Raise the upper body, pointing one elbow towards the opposite knee but keeping your elbows wide. Hold the position as you exhale for seven to ten seconds, imagining that a weight is pressing down heavily on your abdomen.*

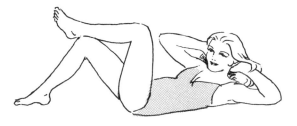

3. *Repeat five times, then repeat another five times with the right heel over the left knee. Finally, repeat the entire sequence two or three times. Note: as the exercise progresses, you may find it difficult to maintain the thought of the weight pressing down on the abdomen; in that case, simply place one or two heavy books on your abdomen.*

Exercise 5:
Pushing Down

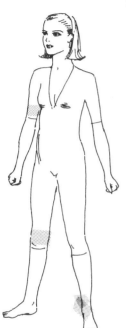

1. *Stand with your legs apart and arms stretched down by your sides. Imagine your feet are pressing 'into' the ground. Breathe in slowly through your nose for seven to ten seconds while clenching your fists and inflating your abdomen as if pushing against a heavy weight.*

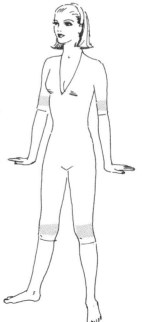

2. *Pause in that position for one or two seconds, then unclench your fists and push your palms down against an imaginary weight while you slowly exhale for seven to ten seconds.*

3. *Repeat five times, pause, then perform the full sequence two or three times over.*

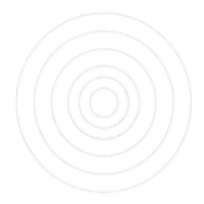

SELF-MASSAGE

MASSAGING YOUR OWN ABDOMEN is a thoroughly natural and instinctive process and is easy to do. In Asia, massage is routinely practised, either at home or together with friends.

Self-massage will help you get to know and respect your abdomen. You will soon discover the key role it plays in terms of digestive disorders, gastric pain, colitis, wind, period pain and constipation. Additionally, you will come to understand how the abdomen can relieve more serious conditions such as type 2 diabetes, unwanted weight gain, cardiovascular disorders, insomnia, fatigue, skin complaints, sexual problems, rheumatism, back pain and many more.

Self-massage induces a sense of well-being at the level of the upper brain by causing the release of endorphins, which are more effective than sedatives in relieving pain.

The small intestine is where nutrients are sorted, processed and channelled via the bloodstream and the lymph glands back into the body as a whole. Its surface comprises between 800 and 900 folds and has around 10 million minuscule villi, which are slender projections from the intestinal mucous membrane. If laid out flat side-by-side, these villi would cover a surface area equivalent to that of a tennis court. Their role is crucial to two-brain equilibrium, as they are linked to the upper brain via the vagus nerve.

Massaging the stomach enhances your powers of concentration; massaging the large intestine reduces emotional stress; massaging the area around the spleen counteracts fatigue and depression; and massaging the liver and bile duct lowers levels of nervous anxiety.

> **Massaging the stomach enhances your powers of concentration; massaging the large intestine reduces emotional stress... around the spleen counteracts fatigue and depression...**

Joëlle was 32 years old when she arrived on my doorstep complaining of fatigue. A local pharmacist had suggested she take vitamin supplements. She had followed his advice but the problem remained: she was still permanently tired and her work was suffering as a result. On examining her, I discovered she was carrying around 5 kilos (11 lbs) of excess weight around her midriff and abdomen. Her abdomen was completely bloated and in spasm, and her solar plexus, gall bladder and pancreas were inflamed. It was clear that Joëlle was eating an excessive amount of sugar-based foods. Blood analysis confirmed as much: with 1.2 grams of sugar in her blood, she was obviously pre-diabetic. What is more, she took no physical exercise whatsoever.

I prescribed abdominal massage each morning and evening, focusing above all on the pancreas. By massaging herself and following the other recommendations in my method (breathing, good nutrition, exercise, meditation), her blood sugar came down to normal (0.8 g) and she shed the unwanted weight.

Massaging the Second Brain

Self-massage is child's play: I should know, because I have practised it since I was very young. There is no need for a special gift, or experience as a professional therapist. Quite the contrary: massaging oneself is straightforward. And the results are more often than not spectacular.

In my book, *Plus jamais mal au dos* ('An End to Back Pain', 2001), I offered advice about self-massaging the lumbar region, neck and shoulders. Thank-you letters poured in, with correspondents expressing their amazement not only at how effective the procedure is but also how easy it is to master. The abdomen is even easier to massage and, because of its direct link to the upper brain, decidedly more receptive to manipulation.

I divide self-massage into two principal groups – calmative self-massage and curative self-massage. Details of both follow.

PART II: THE METHOD

Calmative Self-Massage

Effleurage

The term effleurage *refers to the technique of calmative (i.e. light, soothing and relaxing) massage applied by a clockwise stroking movement of the flat or heel of the hand, in this instance to the entire surface of the abdomen.* Effleurage *utilises barely perceptible pressure and is performed without the use of oils or creams, the intention being to establish maximum direct contact with the skin. It can be practised in the bath or shower. (Total massage time = one minute)*

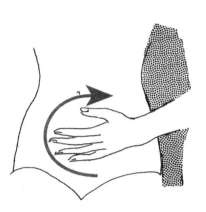

Pressure Massage

Place your hands flat against your abdomen and breathe in to dilate the abdomen while at the same time pressing the hands against it as if trying to prevent it from dilating. Move the hands up and down quickly as you press down. Overall efficacy is enhanced by applying pressure then releasing suddenly. (Total massage time = approximately two minutes)

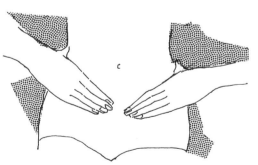

Light Kneading

Working in the breathe-to-relax mode (see pages 46–8), grasp loose abdominal skin in both hands and massage the skin and surrounding tissue as if kneading dough. Palms and fingers should remain in contact with the skin at all times. Hand manipulation should be slow, sustained and without generating friction. (Total massage time = approximately one minute)

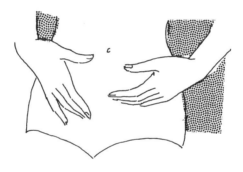

Curative Self-Massage

This category of self-massage is more robust and more precise. You should practise deep abdominal breathing as you work. It focuses on the abdominal plexus and, specifically, on the sensitive pressure points along the meridians which communicate instructions to the body systems, organs and glands. Applying this kind of self-massage requires greater concentration and pressure. No oils or creams are used, and nails should be cut short because you need to use the sensitive tips of the fingers to detect pressure points.

It is important to work on all of these plexuses for a few minutes, two to three times a day. Focus on those that hurt the most when you perform the pinch-and-roll technique (see page 126). Please remember to wait at least two hours after digestion before performing this exercise. When you no longer feel the pain, this indicates that your second brain is cured.

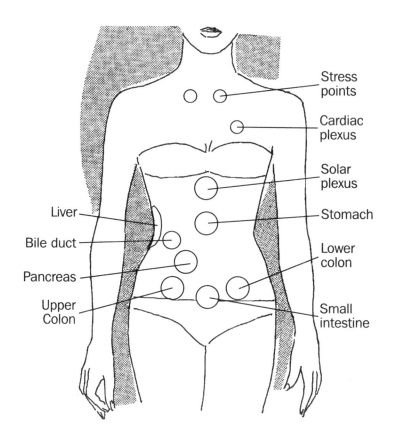

Deep Massage

Use the same techniques as for light massage but work the skin and surrounding tissue more robustly. Deep massage conditions the tissues before you begin the curative self-massage procedures outlined on the previous page. (Total massage time = approximately two minutes)

Pinch-and-Roll

The 'pinch-and-roll' technique involves using one or both hands to grasp an area of skin between the forefinger and thumb and knead the pinched skin between them. This technique is used to disperse cellulite build-up in the connective tissue. Self-massage using the pinch-and-roll technique helps you to find the pressure points that correspond to each system, organ or gland.

If the sites in question are painful, this indicates a dysfunction. The pinch-and-roll procedure is typically accompanied by a very robust kneading motion designed to destroy and eliminate cellulite.

Thirty-five years as a practising therapist have persuaded me that there is no more effective massage or self-massage method for combating cellulite.[28] The technique is actually thousands of years old, pre-dating acupuncture. I used it to 'cure' my own abdomen and I have since recommended it to many others, with similar results. (Total massage time = approximately two to three minutes)

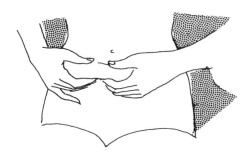

Self-Massaging the Head

Massaging the head can relax the abdomen, thanks to the intimate connection between the two brains.

Sit down and rest your elbows on a table. Use the fingers of both hands to apply a firm massage to the head and scalp, in a circling motion. Include the forehead, the area around the eyebrows, the temples and the nape of the neck. (Total massage time = two to three minutes)

A head massage can be done at any time of day to ease away nervous tension, combat stress, relieve emotional pressures or alleviate fatigue. Massaging the head encourages sleep and stimulating the cranial nerves and part of the vagus nerve helps establish two-brain harmony.

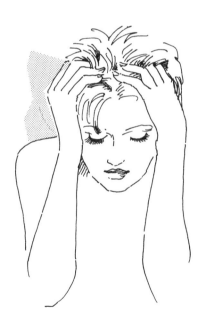

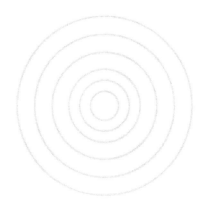

ABDOMINAL MEDITATION

THE ABDOMEN IS A SEPARATE ORGAN that is in communication with the upper brain, generating the vast majority of the body's immune cells and a large number of neuro-transmitters and substances, such as serotonin, which govern our mental state. What this means, in effect, is that a new discipline has come of age: neuro-gastro-enterology.

Recent studies by Professor Gershon and others confirm beyond any reasonable doubt that the abdomen is partially responsible for our emotions. From this point to asserting that we can actually 'think' with our abdomen is only a short step and it is one that I am willing to take without the slightest hesitation.

To my mind, the neurons of the second brain have a life of their own. There are more than 100 million of them – as many as are found in bone marrow – and they produce at least 20 identifiable and autonomous neuro-transmitters identical to those of the upper brain. At INSERM, the Paris-based research institute, a team are at present conducting intensive research into abdominal neutrons and major commercial laboratories are also hard at work in the field, researching new medication. I am persuaded that we will soon be in a position to isolate and define the process of abdominal cell activity in much the same way as we have been proved capable of doing for the upper brain by means of encephalography. What this implies is that treatment for various conditions – such as Alzheimer's – will start with the abdomen.

In the interim, pending the outcome of current research and a full grasp of its practical application, I have developed an abdominal meditation technique designed to complement upper brain activity. In essence, this process will help you 'feel' your abdomen and develop a fuller awareness of how it regulates the 7 metres (23 feet) of digestive tract which house the hypersensitive organisms (villi and micro-villi) that receive and act on messages from the upper brain.

Abdominal meditation is a common practice in the Orient. By focusing on their abdomens, yogis are able to develop total mastery over their behaviour. In some instances, a combination of meditation and deep breathing enables them to alter their blood pressure, reduce or increase their body temperature at will, block or accelerate the digestive process and void their intestines. In India, I was able to observe and analyse these phenom-

PART II: THE METHOD

ena at first hand. There, a healthy abdomen is considered essential for meditation and inner peace. These yogis intuitively sense the harmonious interaction between the two brains and the role performed by the body's neuro-transmitters. For them, as for an increasing number of Westerners, the abdomen is the epicentre of life. I share this view, not least because we now know that childhood experiences (whether happy or sad), hopes, disappointments and all manner of emotional reactions affect the abdomen in much the same way as they affect our upper brain. Recent studies in Canada have convincingly demonstrated that, like the upper brain, the abdomen 'files' our emotions. This kind of research ventures into hitherto virtually unexplored territory, but the implications are enormous, particularly with regard to psychological disorders.

Psychoanalysing the Abdomen

In accordance with the Canadian research mentioned above, I too predict the gradual advent of a fully-fledged psychoanalytical discipline centred on the abdomen. I believe that abdominal meditation, practised in conjunction with abdominal breathing and self-massage, will one day lead to the development of successful treatments for a range of illnesses.[29] As I explained, I succeeded in curing all manner of disorders rooted in my own early childhood, but I found that most of the specialists I talked to were only interested in my upper brain and remained deaf to the complaints emanating from my abdomen.

It took me years to establish that my bodily equilibrium was a function of my two brains working in tandem. My conviction was reinforced by studying Boris Cyrulnik's work on resilience[30], the body's capacity to 'bounce back' in the wake of a traumatic experience. Today, I have not only cured my mind by curing my abdomen, I have also learned to think via the latter. This is the technique I will explain in this section.

Romain, a 27-year-old patient who recently flopped on to my massage table, was very emotional and very timid. He suffered from abdominal pains and admitted to sexual problems. It took me next to no time to trace his condition back to a serious conflict in early childhood. His parents were very strict, there had been a messy divorce and Romain had suffered from depression and sexual inadequacy during his adolescent years. After a few

I believe that abdominal meditation, practised in conjunction with abdominal breathing and self-massage, will lead to the development of treatments for a range of illnesses.

sessions working on his abdomen, I pinpointed painful nodules, which I palpated and massaged. Meanwhile, Romain continued to divulge details of his personal life, uncovering episodes that he had long since forgotten or repressed, such as the sight of his divorced mother in the company of her lover or his own initial sexual 'failure' at the age of seventeen. I used a combination of massage, breathe-to-relax therapy and abdominal meditation. He practised the last of these twice a day. His emotional state became more stable, he re-acquired mastery over his body as a whole and, over several months, he 'rediscovered' his virility. Reconciliation of his two brains had finally opened up the prospects of a happy life.

The Abdominal Meditation Technique

1. *Sit comfortably in an armchair or cross-legged on the floor in a calm, quiet and isolated place conducive to concentration. Place the palms of your hands directly on your abdomen and concentrate on it exclusively. Breathe in deeply and slowly. Your hands should sense a continuous 'burbling' or 'gurgling' sensation that indicates the flow of internal juices.*

2. *Close your eyes and detach yourself as far as possible from your immediate environment, imagining you are in a sort of bubble, deprived of all sensation other than that of touch. Use my breathe-to-relax technique (see page 36) to induce this state. After two to three minutes (perhaps a little longer initially), you will find it helps you shrug off feelings of stress, nervous anxiety and impatience, and you will achieve a condition of receptiveness that is the precursor of abdominal meditation.*

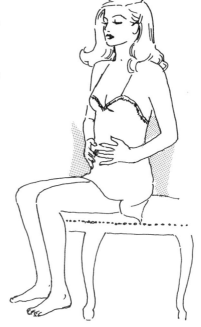

3. *Picture your abdomen as a winding river whose flow may be interrupted by dams, waterfalls, narrows and the like, and whose bed may expand or contract. Fix your mind on these obstacles, which correspond to hard and/or painful points on*

the surface of the abdomen. Then move your hands slowly from the solar plexus (below the breastbone) down and across the entire surface of the abdomen towards the belly.

4. *The meditation process immediately generates a feeling of warmth and will trigger a sense of well-being at the level of the upper brain. Meditation can also help open the floodgates of the unconscious and release memories, emotions and trauma lodged in the lower brain since early childhood. Meditate for ten minutes once or twice daily – or even more, if you feel so inclined. It will probably take you several weeks to progress beyond the initial phase and start to feel your abdomen 'live' under the touch of your hands. As of then, the process of abdominal meditation will become a reality.*

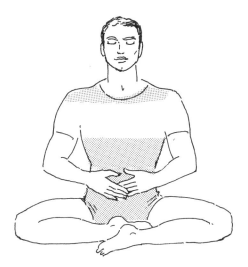

I believe that this abdominal meditation process, which effectively 'recycles' memories from the second brain (the abdomen) to the upper brain, could be the precursor of a new form of analysis or psychotherapy capable of bringing about significant beneficial therapeutic results.

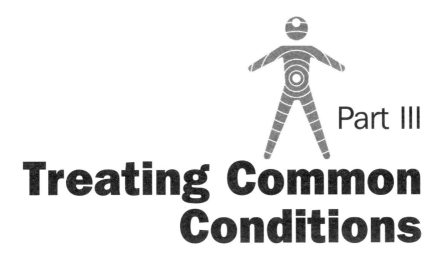

Part III

Treating Common Conditions

In this section I will show you how to use my method to cure some of the common conditions that can make life a misery.

In my view, a disorder occurs when the normal functioning of a system (respiratory, cardiac, nervous or lymphatic), organ, gland, muscle or joint is disrupted. Examples include poor digestion, a distended abdomen, back pain, problems with the circulation in the legs, insomnia, weight gain, sexual problems, anxiety and depression. If these disorders aren't caused by an external aggressor or a fault in the organ, they can be treated and cured.

Even when problems are caused by an illness or infection (such as cardiovascular disease, kidney problems, bacterial or

Creating a healthy equilibrium between abdomen and upper brain will increase the quality and quantity of immune cells. 80 per cent or more of our immune cells are produced in the abdomen.

viral infection, rheumatism, arthritis or tumours), my method can help stabilise a patient's condition, relieving pain and complementing the prescribed course of treatment.

By following my advice and method, you can reduce the risk of a disorder becoming a chronic illness, since creating a healthy equilibrium between abdomen and upper brain will increase the quality and quantity of immune cells. According to some authorities, 80 per cent or more of our immune cells are produced in the abdomen.

Conditions and ailments in this section are listed in alphabetical order. You may need to read more than one. If you suffer from fatigue, insomnia and unwanted weight gain, for example, you should read the advice in all three sections. Few functional disorders exist in isolation. Type 2 diabetes, for example, is almost always linked to weight gain, whereas back pain is often accompanied by sleep disorders, and depression by sexual problems. Note that in this section, the information given under the heading 'Eating' combines advice for the two steps, 'Regular and slow eating' and 'Eating carefully'.

Throughout my career, I have watched patients' functional disorders disappear altogether once they took appropriate action to eliminate abdominal trouble and continued to adhere to my method once overall improvement had set in. That experience underpins the present guide which, I hope, will represent an invaluable aid to your own personal abdominal health.

Ageing

I know from experience that a flabby, protruding abdomen impairs vertebral posture, leading to hunched shoulders and triggering bouts of pessimism and other symptoms of ageing. I have seen men and women in their 30s and 40s who exhibit premature signs of ageing (diminished ambition, fatigue, negativity), but I have also met 70-year-olds who, thanks to a fit abdomen and sound general health, have kept their youthful figure and élan. In the latter cases, a healthy abdomen/upper brain link acts as a catalyst, generating energy and producing immune cells. These 'eternally young' people rarely fall ill; instead, they remain alert, optimistic, open-minded and accessible. What is more, they frequently have a strong sex drive. In other words, they have staved off old age.

PART III: TREATING COMMON CONDITIONS

A flat abdomen is the sign of a well-oxygenated upper brain in full possession of its faculties and a body that has effectively warded off the three major scourges of age – cardiovascular disease, cancer and Alzheimer's.

Eating

It was 2,300 years ago that Hippocrates, the father of medicine, advised: 'Let food be your sole medication.' The risk of digestive disorders increases with age, so what you eat becomes ever more important. First, you should choose what you enjoy, varying your diet and eating slowly, at regular intervals, and in a relaxed state. These measures can help avoid a boredom with food that can lead to a tapering off of the senses of taste and smell and to reduced production of saliva. When the abdomen is deprived of vitamins, essential mineral salts and antioxidants, it can no longer fulfil its function with respect to the immune system and, as a result, will 'disengage' from the upper brain.

The golden rule is: *eat neither too much nor too little, eat only enough*.

Eating *too much* will exhaust the digestive system and cause cholesterol build-up, heart strain, lapses in concentration, elevated blood sugar and unwanted weight gain. The link with the upper brain will be severed. By the same token, eating *too little* can result in hunger pangs, loss of energy, anxiety, depression and frequent infections as the abdomen ceases to generate the requisite amount of immune cells.

Note that the body's calorie requirements do not decrease over time, although if you are less active then you will need to eat less. Otherwise, weight gain or loss could be symptomatic of an impending illness.

Current thinking is that antioxidants are vital for slowing the ageing process. Fruit and vegetables are the primary source of antioxidants, but other sources include phyto-oestrogen hormones (found in soya products and wild yams). Phyto-oestrogens are especially important for women during the menopause.

To offset ageing, eat foods that are as rich as possible in natural vitamins and antioxidants (see pages 87–90). In practice, this means eating dairy products (a pot of yoghurt or a slice of cheese) at least once a day, because the calcium they contain affords protection against osteoporosis. Eat fruit with each meal. Drink between 1 and 2 litres (2–3$^1/_2$ pints) of water daily – more if you are exercising or playing sport. Beware of weight-loss diets, which can exert a negative influence on two-brain harmony and the metabolism as a whole. Any diet intended to eliminate fat will, sadly, also decrease muscle mass which can be difficult to replace.

Remember that sugar-based foods are sworn enemies of the abdomen, with the exception of dark chocolate, of which two squares can be eaten after main meals. Avoid fried foods, cooking in butter, cold meats and spirits and tobacco. On the other hand, feel free to indulge in a glass or two of good wine with a meal.

Many treatments for disease associated with ageing now focus on the abdomen and nutrition. Current research on mice suggests that Alzheimer's can be prevented by a regimen featuring high concentrations of folic acid. Boston's National Institute on Aging conducted trials on 1,000 elderly patients and found that taking folic acid plus vitamins B$_6$ and B$_{12}$ helped them to feel and appear younger. I welcome these developments although I can

PART III: TREATING COMMON CONDITIONS

scarcely keep a smile off my face when I think how often I have treated patients with abdominal complaints and encouraged them to change their eating habits only to be told subsequently that 'everybody says how incredibly young I look now!'

Abdominal Breathing

Abdominal breathing routines eliminate toxins by helping to prevent excessive fermentation in the colon and bowels. It keeps the intestinal mucus healthy, enabling the blood to route nutrients throughout the body and to the upper brain. Abdominal breathing combats ageing since it prevents chronic indigestion, which has a devastating effect on the body's systems, organs and glands. Additionally, it indirectly affects hormone production, including oestrogen in women and DHEA (dehydroepiandrosterone), the now legendary 'fountain of youth' hormone, whose absence reputedly accelerates the ageing process.

Exercises for the Two Brains

The routine on pages 114–19 should be followed twice or three times daily. Muscle mass diminishes with advancing age and it is imperative to maintain it as far as possible in order to protect the joints and avoid rheumatoid complaints and osteoporosis. My two-brain exercise technique affords yet another level of protection against Alzheimer's since it acts on the abdominal cells and the neurons in the upper brain.

Recreational Exercise

Moderate recreational exercise is very important to fortify the cardiovascular system and oxygenate the two brains, thereby inducing both physical and mental relaxation. An American study of over 6,000 women aged over 65 years has demonstrated that walking a mile a day or practising a chosen sport for a period of one hour daily results in a 13 per cent reduction in cognitive decline.

Exercise should be taken three times weekly for a period of at least 45 minutes.

Self-Massage

Finger-massage your gums before every meal and brush your teeth immediately after meals. Between meals, follow my recommendations on abdominal self-massage (pages 120–7), focusing on any areas of discomfort. Self-massage helps to stimulate and fortify the liver, bladder, pancreas, intestine and colon which can become 'lazy' over time.

Abdominal Meditation

Abdominal meditation is increasingly necessary as you age. In the first instance, it helps develop a serene outlook and a respect for life. By practising abdominal meditation, you will learn (or re-learn) how to be content, optimistic, happy and caring; conversely, it will be help to counteract stress and depression and, according to Professor Snowdon of the University of Kentucky, meditation will add ten years to your life.

Anxiety and Nervous Tension

The abdomen is the seat of emotional stresses such as shyness, lack of self-confidence, hypersensitivity and anxiety.[31] These emotional states are perceived in the upper brain and replicated in the abdomen; by the same token, any abdominal malfunction or disorder is transmuted into emotion at the level of the upper brain. Discovery of the key role played by the cranial nerves (linked to the abdomen via the vagus nerve) and heightened awareness of the importance of two-way neuro-transmitters have confirmed the importance of the abdomen in causing psychological disorders of all kinds.

Caring for the abdomen can help eradicate fears, anxieties and complexes which extend back into early childhood. Stress and strong emotional pressures disrupt our body clock and we tend to compensate by eating more – typically 'comfort food'. Alternatively, we may stop eating. This is clearly harmful to the

> **Stress and strong emotional pressures disrupt our body clock and we tend to compensate by eating more – typically 'comfort food'... This is clearly harmful to the abdomen...**

abdomen and, by extension, the upper brain. The side effects are well known: disrupted sleep patterns, lowered morale and sexual impotence in men, frigidity in women. In such cases, our susceptibility to allergies intensifies; there is often unwanted weight gain or weight loss and nervous tension increases, frequently to the point of severe depression.

Abdominal Breathing

Abdominal deep breathing can effectively neutralise the anxieties and depression caused by profound emotional stress.

When the first symptoms of stress appear, follow my breathe-to-relax sequence (see pages 46–8) five times, then start again, breathing even more deeply and gently. Each time you breathe out from your abdomen, imagine that you are breathing out the anxiety from your system, in a method I call the 'anti-stress filter'. Repeat several times every day. We now know that stress can cause acute abdominal discomfort, including diarrhoea. My breathing method will counteract these and similar malfunctions and eliminate stress at the level of the upper brain.

Eating

A study involving 1,000 inmates in a number of US penitentiaries established that aggressive behaviour and anxieties can be mitigated by reducing sugar intake, acid foods and red meat, so it can be a good idea to try this if you are feeling anxious.

My other advice to those who suffer from anxiety is as follows:

• Eat an antacid breakfast every morning (see pages 92–3) and be sure to eat slowly; anxiety levels rise when you eat too quickly.
• Avoid structured weight-loss diets, since the abdomen and the central nervous system respond negatively to fasting.
• Never skip a meal. In fact, you should complement your regular meals with small mid-morning or mid-afternoon snacks.

Exercises for the Two Brains

Two-brain exercises can be a powerful antidote to anxiety and stress by balancing the upper brain, breathing and abdomen. This will restore inner balance and harmony after only a few sessions. However, if practised too vigorously, too quickly or in an inappropriate environment, two-brain exercises may provoke psychological and physiological dislocation (which typically manifests itself as abnormal perspiration). If practised as described on pages 114–19, however, it will prove beneficial and effective. Two-brain exercises should be performed at least twice daily.

Recreational Exercise

Exercise is a great method of relieving anxieties and tensions. Exercise for at least 45 minutes at a time, three times a week. This will help you relax, sharpen your senses and think positively, and it will be even more beneficial if performed outdoors. There will be a calmative effect on the upper brain, which will be in tune with your abdomen.

Self-Massage

Abdominal massage, whether performed by yourself or by others will immediately calm the two brains and reduce tension and anxiety levels. Self-massage may include forceful palpation of the various abdominal plexuses (see page 124). Abdominal massage can be alternated with head massage (see page 127). In every instance, the massage should be synchronised with abdominal breathing patterns.

Abdominal Meditation

Perform daily meditation sessions with your hands on your abdomen (see pages 132–3). As you breathe in and out calmly and deeply, energy can be channelled to the upper brain. Imagine the energy extending in soothing waves throughout your whole body. Direct it first to the head, then to the back, the chest, the arms and the legs, then 'think' it back once again to the abdomen.

Asthma and Respiratory Disease

Evidence laid before the most recent World Congress of Pneumology detailed the risks and benefits to lungs and bronchial tubes of certain foodstuffs. Asthma, rhinitis and ear-nose-and-throat infections caused by chemical pollutants, central heating, air-conditioning, mould, mites, pollen and animal hair are closely linked to food intake and the central nervous system (upper brain). It is now accepted that acute stress can provoke or exacerbate asthma, as can tobacco (particularly in women, whose lung capacity is less than that of their male counterparts) or an excess of alcohol.

By targeting chronic indigestion and reinforcing the intestinal flora, I have frequently been able to alleviate or even cure rhinitis, sinusitis, inflammation of the throat and ear infections, and ward off asthma attacks. What is more, I have achieved excellent longer-term results by persuading patients to adopt my seven-point method on an ongoing basis.

Asthma is one of the most common ailments among young children. In my experience, various problems experienced by asthma sufferers arise as a direct consequence of consuming sugary snacks (drinks, biscuits, sweets) but these can be alleviated by substituting wholemeal bread sandwiches and fresh fruit. The incidence of asthma attacks will decrease, as will recourse to medication prescribed to avert those attacks.

Eating

Respiratory insufficiency can almost without exception be sourced to nutrient deficiency. To boost the respiratory function, it is important to remember the following:

PART III: TREATING COMMON CONDITIONS

- Eat slowly, at regular intervals and in calm surroundings. Teenagers who skip meals or clandestinely snack on sugar-based foods exhibit a much higher incidence of respiratory troubles.
- Avoid foods that can cause bloating or are disruptive to the digestive system in any way, including fish preserved in oil, soya products, milk chocolate, peanuts and peanut oil, dairy products, eggs, seafood, melted cheese, fried butter, white flour and dried fruits.
- Opt instead for foods with protective qualities, such as green vegetables and fresh fruit. Research carried out in the United Kingdom has recently highlighted the beneficial effects of apples, noting that eating five a week increases the respiratory volume by some 140 ml.

Abdominal Breathing

Deep abdominal breathing causes expansion of the ribcage and strengthens the respiratory muscles. Additionally, it stimulates the development of blood vessels in the nasal passages that can help to filter out impurities. This is especially true in post-menopausal women, who are more prone to asthma than men.

By soothing the nervous system, abdominal breathing combats nervous tension, timidity and the hypersensitivity that is one of the causes of respiratory problems. If possible, the abdominal breathing routine should be followed five times an hour (see pages 36–48).

Recreational Exercise

Exercise is a tried-and-tested ally in the battle against asthma and other respiratory disorders. It reinforces the cardiovascular system, stimulates and strengthens glands and organs, expels toxins and boosts the immune system. Asthmatics should avoid exercise that is too strenuous, as training to excess can lead to a respiratory insufficiency, particularly in the absence of inadequate warm-up and recovery times. In those instances, the answer is to reduce the effort or pace involved rather than cut out exercise entirely. The best types of exercise for those with respiratory disorders are swimming, walking and hiking.

Exercises for the Two Brains

By strengthening the abdominal muscles, two-brain exercises eliminate excess stomach acids that cause chronic indigestion, which, according to the World Congress of Pneumology, can cause respiratory problems. An abdomen that is distended, bloated and in spasm is, quite simply, a repository for breathing disorders.

Self-Massage

Massaging the abdomen and chest relaxes the upper brain, stimulates the plexus and meridians, and releases energies that are invaluable in combating respiratory problems.

Abdominal Meditation

This technique (see pages 128–33) can help alleviate the symptoms of breathlessness and fatigue characteristic of an asthma attack.

Back Pain, Arthritis and Rheumatism

Strange as it may at first seem, successful treatment of back pain is first and foremost a matter of caring for the abdomen. In my book *Plus jamais mal au dos* ('An End to Back Pain'), I

explained that when a patient complains of back pain, I immediately examine his or her abdomen. A distended abdomen
will place strain on the back and affect the posture. Palpating
the abdomen will almost invariably reveal that it is bloated
and in spasm, with hyperacidity affecting the muscles and
joints. Many back and rheumatic complaints can be traced
directly to the abdomen. Spanish physician Ramôn y Cajal
postulates that 'interstitial' cells (those that fill gaps between
tissues) produced by the abdomen play an important part in
the proper functioning of the muscles by 'relaying' messages
from the upper brain. (This does not apply, of course, in the

> **...when a patient complains of back pain, I
> immediately examine his or her abdomen. A
> distended abdomen will place strain on the
> back and affect the posture.**

case of back complaints stemming from a fall or other such
trauma.)

Abdominal acidity causes inflammation of the intestinal
mucus, reduces muscle flexibility and blocks spinal and joint
articulation. As a result, it is the most frequent cause of back
and rheumatic problems. The standard reaction is to prescribe
anti-inflammatory medication, often in escalating doses, but this
has implications for the digestive system, as analgesics can cause
gastritis and ulcers. By exacerbating hyperacidity, they also give
rise to all manner of digestive problems, causing increased
fatigue and, when the treatment is eventually discontinued,
may result in depression caused by recurrent pain. By contrast,

an antacid treatment coupled with relaxation of the central nervous system by means of two-brain exercises, appropriate recreational exercise and self-massage can prove effective in the majority of cases of recurrent or chronic back or joint pain.

Eating
- Eat an antacid breakfast (see pages 92–3).
- Divide daily food intake into five light and varied meals, and eat slowly.
- Avoid acid foods, which are liable to cause intestinal fermentation and related digestive problems. Excessive acid intake can have a negative impact on joints and can cause pain. In particular, avoid taking coffee, tea, alcohol, tobacco or fruit juices on an empty stomach. A US research study involving 30,000 subjects who drank at least four cups of coffee a day revealed that the incidence of rheumatoid polyarthritis was significantly higher in coffee-drinkers than non-coffee-drinkers. Drinking decaffeinated coffee did not substantially affect these findings.
- You should also avoid honey, jams, white-flour pastries, pizzas, quiches, biscuits, white bread and melted cheese.
- Avoid sugary drinks (fizzy or non-fizzy).
- Limit your intake of red meat, cold meats and fried foods.
- Avoid cooking with butter or cooking fats.

To sum up: opt as far as possible for an alkaline diet (raw or cooked green vegetables, potatoes, corn, cabbage, carrots, beetroot, green beans, spinach) with lots of aromatic herbs with antioxidant properties (chives, parsley, basil, tarragon) and fruits and nuts (bananas, peaches, chestnuts, almonds). White meat, notably veal and poultry (chicken, guinea fowl, turkey), are recommended.

PART III: TREATING COMMON CONDITIONS

Pasta, rice, broad beans, lentils, fava beans, and low-GI foods (see page 79) help to protect the back and joints.

Recreational Exercise

Moderate physical activity on a regular basis is recommended by most medical specialists as an excellent means of counteracting and reducing inflammation, relieving aches and pains and preserving muscle tone. The aim is to strengthen the joints without causing pain or swelling. You should avoid strenuous or rapid movements, or those that place too great a strain on the joints.

To combat back pain and rheumatic discomfort, it is important to get to know your own body and recognise its limits. This takes time and patience. I agree with Professor Xavier Chevalier of the Henri-Mondor Hospital in Créteil, who stresses that 'a non-pharmacological approach is a first and indispensable step in the treatment of arthritis in terms of ameliorating not only physical function but also reducing the threshold of pain'.

Recreational exercises most conducive to developing a healthy back and averting rheumatic discomfort include the following:

Swimming in moderation. Swimming does not place undue strain on the joints. What is more, warm water – preferably salt water – is beneficial so long as you don't spend too much time in it. Swimming gently for, say, 20 minutes should suffice. Aqua-aerobics are a great idea and your local pool may have classes or guided sessions available.

Cycling is recommended, provided that the terrain is relatively flat and that care is taken to get a saddle of the right height and position for your physique. Avoid over-exertion and take a break every 30 minutes or so, during which gentle stretching exercises are a good idea. If, for one reason or another, you are unable to cycle outdoors, an exercise bicycle may be substituted.

Walking is also highly recommended. Wear walking shoes with cushioned soles to prevent strain on the Achilles tendon. Wear light clothes (a heavy jacket will exacerbate inflammation if you suffer from lumbar or cervical degeneration). Do not carry a shoulder bag, since this imbalances the body. Stop for a rest every 20 minutes or so.

Exercising gently and at regular intervals helps to relax the central nervous system, stabilises body weight, strengthens the joints and restores abdominal health. Remember to drink water

> **Exercising gently and at regular intervals helps to relax the central nervous system, stabilises body weight, strengthens the joints and restores abdominal health.**

before, during and after physical exercise.

Exercises for the Two Brains

These are particularly recommended in cases of back pain or rheumatism, and won't cause any additional strain on muscles and joints (see pages 108–19).

Abdominal Breathing

My breathing recommendations are designed to promote increased blood flow and to eliminate unwanted acid deposits accumulated as a result of excessive intestinal fermentation affecting the muscles and joints (see pages 36–48).

Self-Massage

My method of abdominal self-massage is risk-free. It will help to eliminate digestive disorders and reduce excessive abdominal acidity, which impacts on the joints. A self-massage routine should be followed two or three times daily (see pages 120–7).

Abdominal Meditation

Back pain and rheumatism are particularly responsive to the sense of relaxation generated by establishing and sustaining two-brain harmony (see pages 128–33).

Cancer

It is now accepted that immune system deficiency is one of the factors that can lead to the growth of cancerous tumours. At a conservative estimate, the abdomen produces 80 per cent of the body's immune cells. Accordingly, I cannot stress enough the importance of the abdomen's role in the fight against cancer, both in preventing the onset and in curing cancer. Today, statistics indicate that in the Western world more than 50 per cent of all cancers respond positively to treatment. On countless occasions over the years, I have worked on the abdomens of cancer patients and found that they were distended, rigid and painful. I tried to alleviate the patient's discomfort and suffering and, by boosting morale, help him or her through the thoroughly unpleasant processes of chemotherapy, radiation or surgery.

I am convinced that if in future we develop a closer relationship between medical treatments and abdominal care, we will achieve even more positive results in the battle against cancer.

Eating

There are literally thousands of studies and scientific research papers devoted to the role of the abdomen and nutrition in the treatment of cancer. It is now generally acknowledged that roughly 30 per cent of cancer cases in the developed world are linked to nutritional factors; a 2001 Europe-wide EPIC (European Prospective Investigation into Cancer) study spearheaded by Dr Riboldi would appear to substantiate this.[32]

For my own part, I am persuaded that a diversified food intake rich in antioxidant fruits and vegetables (see pages 87–9) will reduce the risks of cancer. More specifically, I advise that you

> **...if in future we develop a closer relationship between medical treatments and abdominal care, we will achieve even more positive results in the battle against cancer.**

avoid the following:

- foods containing free radicals that cause oxidation, notably barbecued meat, fish, sausages and potatoes; Montpellier-based cancer specialist Professor Henri Joyeux is of the opinion that 'a barbecued steak has the same carcinogenic impact as smoking one thousand cigarettes'
- recycled oils, fried butter, and over-ripe fruit with mould or traces of pesticide
- foods containing white flour, including white bread, pizzas, cakes and certain breakfast cereals
- dairy products (an excessive calcium intake destroys vitamin D);

however, goat's cheese can be eaten occasionally because it is less fatty than other cheeses

• all food additives.

To reduce the risk of cancer, make sure your diet includes soya, broccoli, endive, celery, rice, sesame seeds, chickpeas, fava beans, dark chocolate and plenty of antioxidants (see pages 87, 88 and 89).

Abdominal Breathing

My abdominal breathing approach (see pages 36–48) helps to stimulate the circulation of the blood and, in consequence, encourage the formation of immune cells in the abdomen. This, in tandem with the upper brain, induces mental relaxation which, in turn, aids cancer prevention. Abdominal breathing helps eliminate toxins more rapidly and may, in my opinion, retard the progress of cancer.

Self-Massage

Gentle massage can help to make the abdomen more flexible and less prone to cramps, thus improving the condition of the digestive system as a whole.

Recreational Exercise

Playing sport can help cancer patients overcome the depression which typically sets in, and can combat a potential weakening of the digestive system and muscles. Cancer always brings a feeling of general lassitude and fatigue, so any recreational exercise must be taken in moderation. Nevertheless, it can be valuable in boosting the body's immuno-defensive system as a whole.

Abdominal Meditation

This procedure, described in detail on pages 128–33, can help to improve the state of mind. Some specialists believe that a positive mental attitude can cause cancers to regress or even disappear. I think that concentrating on the abdomen can be an important factor in the successful treatment of cancer.

Cardiovascular Disorders

Ever since I started practising as a healer, I have insisted that focusing on abdominal health will make a major contribution to the treatment of serious cardiovascular disorders. In most instances, these develop as a result of deposits of bad cholesterol, inordinately high blood sugar levels (diabetes) or a general 'clogging' of the circulatory system. These aggressive conditions can all be traced back to the abdomen.

There is a tendency to treat the heart only when it is directly under threat. Great strides have been taken in this respect[33] but much remains to be accomplished, not least in terms of underlining the importance of the close interrelationship that persists between the upper and lower brains. An unhealthy abdomen and chronic indigestion stemming from deficient intestinal flora exert undue strain on the circulatory system, whose task it is to convey blood to the mucous membranes in order to offset inflammation. This, in turn, results in progressive acceleration of cardiac rhythms, leading to breathlessness, chest pain, headaches, depression and other 'upper brain' disorders.

To put it another way, the link between upper brain and heart passes via the abdomen. It has recently been established that a neuro-transmitter produced in the abdomen – known as

PART III: TREATING COMMON CONDITIONS

neurotrophine – plays a pivotal role in regulating blood pressure. I have frequently given a new lease on life to patients with cardiac problems by helping to alleviate abnormally high or abnormally low blood pressure.

Abdominal Breathing
Abdominal breathing (see pages 36–48), by improving oxygenation of the entire body and expanding the ribcage, tones and protects the heart muscle and bolsters the cardiovascular system as a whole. Additionally, it helps limit stress by increasing the output of serotonin. In women, stress reduces oestrogen levels, thereby depriving the body of its natural protection.

Eating
The importance of choosing your foods carefully, combined with eating slowly, in moderation and at regular intervals (see pages 49–69), is confirmed by a recent study (conducted by the Silvia Titan Group in Cambridge) involving 15,000 subjects aged between 45 and 75 years. The study reported a significant lowering of total and LDL cholesterol levels as a result of an antioxidant-based regimen (see pages 87–9). Subjects ate meals with plenty of fruit, vegetables and fibre, while avoiding rich, fatty or sugary foodstuffs which can cause obesity and diabetes and induce an excess of blood flow to the abdomen. This is my primary dietary advice for everyone, not just those with existing cardiovascular problems.

Tobacco destroys the majority of antioxidant vitamins generated by the abdomen (above all, Vitamin C), increases the risk of cardiovascular disease by hardening the arteries (including the aorta, which runs through the abdomen), and generating cholesterol build-up on the inner surfaces of the arteries (atheroma). Wine contains certain antioxidants (tannins and flavonoids) and I recommend one glass (or, at the very most, two) to accompany a meal; at the same time, I recommend that you avoid drinking before or after a meal. A cup of green or black tea taken mid-morning or mid-afternoon will have an antioxidant effect.

Recreational Exercise

Regular and moderate exercise helps maintain a healthy abdomen (see pages 98–107) and has a positive impact in the battle against atherosclerosis, the principal cause of cardiovascular malfunction. The American Heart Association confirmed as much at its most recent congress: 'Regular low-intensity physical exercise, such as walking four or five times a week, lowers reactive protein C blood level content and enhances the action of cells coating the blood-vessels. This is particularly noted in the case of males, who have a more pronounced genetic predisposition to cardiovascular disorders.'[34]

Self-Massage

Massage – and particularly abdominal massage – is beneficial because it stimulates oxygenation of the circulatory system and, by interacting with the upper brain, induces relaxation. It's also useful to self-massage your chest and head (see pages 120–7). Massaging the chest effectively massages the heart, thereby improving abdominal blood flow and facilitating the digestive process.

Abdominal Meditation

Abdominal meditation reduces stress and diminishes cardiovascular risk. An in-depth study by the US National Institute of Health has recently postulated that meditation, which enables an individual to project himself into a spiritual dimension, lowers the risk of stroke and heart attacks (see pages 132–3).

Cellulite

Cellulite has its origins in the abdomen. It follows that the only means of combating cellulite is to restore health to the abdomen and, at the same time, to promote upper brain relaxation.

> **...the only means of combating cellulite is to restore health to the abdomen and, at the same time, to promote upper brain relaxation.**

Cellulite is more common in women, and occurs most noticeably around the waistline, the buttocks, the thighs and on the upper arms. In men, it tends to be in the abdomen or around the neck. Cellulite is not necessarily a condition brought on by being overweight and slimming may not result in its disappearance; instead, it is always a result of a deregulated nervous system impacting negatively on the digestive process and causing a constant excess of fermentation in the gut. This, in turn, results in toxins being retained and leads to chronic 'intoxication' in the broadest sense of that term. As blood pumps through the abdomen, it extracts not only valuable nutrients but also toxins, which are then deposited in certain areas of the body. The result is cellulite build-up, accompanied almost invariably by a dislocation of the upper brain causing nervous anxiety and irritability.

All anti-cellulite 'miracle cures' (for example, injections, infiltration, liposuction, lymphatic drainage, laser treatment or 'slimming' creams) are, in my view, ineffectual and, at times, positively dangerous.

Eating

Food intake is important if you want to beat cellulite. As usual, eat slowly and in calm surroundings. On no account should you skip meals. You should also avoid snacking between meals, since this disrupts the proper functioning of the kidneys, the bile duct and the pancreatic tract. Formal dieting should, to my mind, never be a long-term option.

My first objective is to calm the upper brain, initially by reassuring the patient. I have effected some quite remarkable results without any huge changes in diet. I simply ask patients to reduce the quantity of high-risk foods and drinks and change the order in which they eat foods during the day. This approach prevents a sense of frustration at the level of the upper brain, a condition which is harmful to abdominal health. According to my experience there are three types of candidates susceptible to cellulite build-up:

- Sugar and pastry addicts. Don't cut these out entirely but reduce your intake by half.
- 'Foodies': feel free to eat out in restaurants but take care to eat in moderation and only when you are hungry.
- Those who cannot exist without coffee, tea, alcohol or tobacco. My advice is to learn to savour and appreciate, while progressively reducing the quantities consumed. This will help relax the

upper brain. For example: only drink coffee after eating something solid and restrict yourself to a single glass of wine a day.

Abdominal Breathing

Relaxing the upper brain by practising abdominal breathing makes it easier to stand back and take stock. This will increase your overall energy levels and enable you to reduce the quantities of food you eat, reduce the fermentation process and, over time, eliminate cellulite (see pages 36–48).

Recreational Exercise

Exercise calms the upper brain and stimulates various processes in the human body, notably the cardiovascular, digestive and lymphatic systems. There will also be improved circulation, which will help to eliminate toxins. Cellulite cannot be treated successfully if you don't do some form of endurance sport (see page 100) at least twice or three times a week, for a minimum of 45 minutes at a time.

Exercises for the Two Brains

The aim is to 'sculpt' the body as a whole and to improve the muscle tone and overall condition of the abdomen. Daily two-brain exercises will destroy cellulite in time (see pages 108–19).

Self-Massage

This will help you to locate and break up the major cellulite deposits in your abdomen. Once the abdominal deposits have been removed, cellulite deposits elsewhere – on the buttocks, thighs and arms – will disappear rapidly (see pages 120–7).

Abdominal Meditation

It's important to relax your upper brain in order to combat cellulite and unwanted weight gain. Abdominal meditation fosters relaxation by harmonising the two brains (see pages 128–33).

Colitis, Crohn's Disease and Irritable Bowel Syndrome

Colitis – inflammation of the colon – Crohn's Disease and irritable bowel syndrome (IBS) are all common intestinal conditions that frequently result from poor eating habits. They can be aggravated by stress, anxiety, nervous tension, emotional pressures or general hypersensitivity.

Colitis attacks the intestinal lining and opens the door to agents which cause functional disorders and illnesses. Symptoms can include painful cramps, wind, fatigue and, more often than not, constipation, as well as an overall sense of exhaustion and irascibility. Colitis, Crohn's and IBS all attest to a lack of equilibrium between the two brains.

Intestinal problems diminish immunity and cause persistent fermentation of food in the intestine, retarding the absorption–elimination process and, in the longer term, leading to chronic indigestion. The intestines can be described as a sinuous path with occasional hairpin bends. When food ferments in one of these bends, it lodges there for longer than normal and triggers irritation of the mucous membrane which, in turn, infects other parts of the intestinal tract. Strenuous physical activity or emotional stress cause the folds and bends to constrict and disrupt the digestive process as a whole.

In practical terms, this means that the digestive process, which normally takes around three hours, can effectively double, resulting in fatigue, constipation and the formation of cellulite. As blood pumps through the intestinal tract it extracts not only valuable nutrients such as vitamins, mineral salts and trace elements, but it also absorbs infectious agents that can poison glands and organs (such as the liver and kidneys). Where a patient has a predisposition towards rheumatism, increased inflammation of the joints may also occur.

Curing colitis, Crohn's and IBS is relatively simple, provided that you make changes in your eating habits and learn to modify your body clock to relax and achieve two-brain harmony. [35]

Breathing patterns directly affect colitis, Crohn's and IBS because relaxing the upper brain has a calmative effect on the abdomen.

Abdominal Breathing

Breathing patterns directly affect colitis, Crohn's and IBS because relaxing the upper brain has a calmative effect on the abdomen. Before sitting down to eat – and at all times when you feel stressed or otherwise out of sorts – follow my breathe-to-relax method (see pages 46–8).

Exercises for the Two Brains

I advise against straining the abdominal muscles when the intestines are already inflamed. This intensifies colonic response and may either cause or further aggravate a pre-existing hiatus (stomach) or groin hernia.

Consult my recommendations for light two-brain exercises (see pages 112–9) and select those movements that involve exerting pressure on the abdomen. As soon as the problem has disappeared, start exercising the abdominal muscles again in order to energise the system as a whole and, in the process, develop a flat abdomen.

Eating

In a nutshell:

- Avoid eating large meals and eating too quickly, since insufficient chewing is one of the root causes of colitis, Crohn's and IBS.
- Never skip breakfast but opt instead for a light first meal of the day (see pages 94–95). The stomach secretes extremely potent gastric juices at regular intervals – three times daily if you eat three meals a day – and, if those juices have nothing to work on, they will attack the stomach wall, disrupting the bile, pancreatic and pylorus tracts, provoking abnormal fermentation in the intestines which, over time, can develop into colitis.
- Avoid stimulants taken on an empty stomach, especially tea and coffee (with or without milk), dried apricots and prunes, beer, cider, sugary drinks and fruit juice. Avoid also fried foods, pimentos, harissa (a spicy Middle Eastern paste) and spicy foods generally, together with any foods that cause bloating (soups, dishes with sauces, pastries). Not least, moderate your intake of cold meats, fried butter, white bread, breadcrumbs, biscuits and melted cheese.
- Sip mineral water (2 litres/3$^1/_2$ pints) daily) and/or infusions of verbena, rosemary and other herbal teas.
- Never sit down to eat while in a disturbed emotional state.

PART III: TREATING COMMON CONDITIONS

Recreational Exercise

Practising moderate endurance sports on a regular basis combats and eliminates excess fermentation and helps cure colitis, Crohn's and IBS. But note the following:

• Extreme sports accelerate intestinal fermentation and lead to cramps.
• When out walking, stride rather than step.
• After swimming, wrap up well to preclude abdominal chills.

Self-Massage

Massage the abdomen twice daily between meals, focusing on the small intestine pressure point situated below the navel and the upper and lower colon (see pages 124–5).

Abdominal Meditation

Abdominal meditation (see pages 128–33) enables you to identify pains and cramps caused by colitis, Crohn's and IBS that may be a result of early childhood trauma or residual emotional stress. After a while, you will begin to feel relief from some of your symptoms and you will sense your abdomen coming to life again.

Constipation

The causes of constipation are too numerous and diverse to be listed here. Some are purely physical, notably when the intestine walls are attacked by acids due to excessive fermentation or dehydration of the stool. Other causes stem from the upper brain and are a consequence of early childhood fears and trauma as well as the pressures of modern everyday life. A sedentary lifestyle, poor time management, irregular eating patterns and certain weight-loss diets frequently result in constipation and its typical corollary: haemorrhoids ('piles').

My seven-step method has never failed to relieve constipation in all of my 35 years as a therapist.

Abdominal Breathing

Learning to relax is a prerequisite of curing constipation. My abdominal breathing approach (see pages 36–48) should be followed on a regular basis if you are nervous or stressed, in order to harmonise the upper and lower brains.

Exercises for the Two Brains

Constipation invariably leads to a swollen and distended abdomen. By restoring the abdomen to full health, constipation can be cured and a flat belly achieved. To this end, exercise your abdominal muscles for three or four minutes at a time, ideally in the early morning and in the evening (see pages 112–9). Exercise in moderation and avoid placing too great a strain on the muscles.

Eating

• Never breakfast in bed; instead, get up as soon as you are awake in order to stimulate the kidney and bile functions.
• Breakfast lightly (see pages 94–5) and, more importantly, slowly and in quiet surroundings. After eating something solid, drink my recommended cocktail of freshly squeezed fruit juices: $1/_3$ orange juice, $1/_3$ grapefruit juice and $1/_3$ lemon juice. Once constipation has been treated, opt instead for a piece of fresh seasonal fruit; this will prove more readily digestible than fruit

juice. Halfway through breakfast, take a teaspoonful of olive oil. A small cup of coffee or tea after a meal helps the digestion and the elimination process, but a large quantity of black coffee or several cups of tea on an empty stomach will have the reverse effect.

- Drink at least 1½ litres (2½ pints) of liquids a day in the form of mineral water, clear vegetable broth or soothing herbal infusions.
- Be wary of laxatives; these irritate the mucous membrane and encourage or intensify intestinal sluggishness, resulting over time in the loss of trace elements and/or mineral salts.

Movement is essential, because sedentary occupations and lifestyles result in 'lazy' intestines and are not conducive to regular bowel movements.

- Laxative suppositories are artificial lubricants and, as such, cause dryness in the intestinal mucus, effectively stopping the natural process of evacuation.
- Avoid excess in all things: sugar-based foods, honey, jams, pastries, white flour (including white bread, biscuits, quiches, pizzas), fried foods, fried butter, cold meats and melted cheese.
- Eat moderate quantities of cooked or raw fibre-rich green vegetables at regular intervals (see page 78).
- Note that an excess of raw vegetables and fruit will supply too much fibre which, in turn, could irritate the mucous membrane and trigger undue fermentation, causing constipation.
- Avoid fibre-rich 'diet' foods (high-bran bread, cereal bars,

lozenges and so on). Not only will they fail to achieve the desired effect, but they will also cause flatulence.

• Eat small meals to avoid overloading the kidneys.

Recreational Exercise

Walk for one hour or two half-hours daily, taking large strides as you do so, or practise an endurance sport of your choice (see page 101). Movement is essential, because sedentary occupations and lifestyles result in 'lazy' intestines and are not conducive to regular bowel movements.

Self-Massage

• After a light breakfast, brush your teeth and finger-massage your gums for two minutes. This will help relax your central nervous system (upper brain), which will promote a healthy abdomen (second brain) and a positive interaction between the two.

• Visit the toilet after breakfast even if you feel no immediate need for a bowel movement.

• Massage your abdomen lightly or deeply in a clockwise direction, kneading the skin and surrounding tissue to eliminate abdominal cellulite build-up. Do this for two to three minutes at a time, once before breakfast and once again before dinner (see pages 120–7).

Depression

Depression is first and foremost a state of mind, but it is also an abdominal condition. There is incontrovertible scientific evidence pointing to the fact that there is a symbiotic relationship between our two brains as a result of reciprocal influences

PART III: TREATING COMMON CONDITIONS

carried by the vagus nerve, supported by a complex system of neuro-transmitters and interstitial cells. This relationship is at its most evident in the case of depression, when a person is 'down' and everything seems somehow 'wrong'. The outer signs of this depression are familiar: lapses in concentration, anxiety, melancholy and maybe sudden fits of aggression. Adolescents are particularly prone to this condition, which can sometimes be accompanied by anorexia or bulimia.

When the upper brain is distressed, the abdomen suffers; conversely, when there is abdominal pain, the upper brain is immediately responsive. Disappointments, disagreements or any

Negative thoughts weigh heavily on the abdomen and disrupt its proper functioning. The body is isolated from the mind and the rupture between the two brains is total.

form of emotional upheaval will 'tie the abdomen in knots'. Equally, a disruption of the digestive process will affect the upper brain. Once the two brains start working in harmony, however, the symbiosis is total and the entire body operates as a single unit.

Depression is frequently accompanied by sexual problems, chest pains, headaches, weight problems and a general feeling of fatigue. Negative thoughts weigh heavily on the abdomen and disrupt its proper functioning. The body is isolated from the mind and the rupture between the two brains is total. Left to its own devices, the abdomen responds by malfunctioning. The first priority is to restore it to health and to address the depression by restoring equilibrium between the two brains. To my mind, we are on the brink of a new form of psychotherapy, which regards the upper brain and abdomen as an ensemble. A primary effect of such an approach would be to limit the intake of anti-depressants.

Eating

Nutrients modify the brain chemistry in ways that are exceedingly complex and not yet fully understood. I believe that if we are prepared to eat sensibly and avoid fatty and sugary foods, we can enhance our own sense of well-being.

Serotonin and noradrenaline are key substances that regulate our food intake. Depression can induce anarchic eating habits in some people, whereas in others it results in the appetite being reduced at times to the point of anorexia.

Certain foods are natural anti-depressants as they contain amino acids that persuade the neuro-transmitters to transmit a peaceful and relaxed state of mind.

Points to remember:

• Carbohydrates have a role to play in alleviating depression. They calm the body down and impart a sense of well-being. That said, it's better to opt for pasta, rice, wholegrain bread, vegetables and fruits than pastries, cakes and biscuits, which could make you put on weight.

• Fats can be pleasurable to eat, but too much fatty food results in lapses in concentration and drowsiness after meals.

• Wholegrain cereals, green vegetables and fresh fruit, certain mineral waters and dark chocolate are beneficial for their high magnesium content.

- Selenium is an indispensable trace element found in eggs, seafood, nuts, dairy produce, white meat and poultry.
- Calcium is a natural tranquillizer and also a mood-enhancer. It is present in milk, cheese, yoghurt, fresh butter, eggs, spinach, almonds, tofu, fish (whitebait, sardines and canned salmon, eaten with bones), shellfish and certain mineral waters.
- Vitamin B_6 is also an effective ally in the battle against depression. It is present in wholegrain cereals, bananas, fish, green vegetables and lean meat.

Recreational Exercise

A team of UK researchers writing in the *British Journal of Sports Medicine* advanced the hypothesis that physical exercise has a powerful anti-depressant effect. According to their studies, it increases the body's output of phenylethylamine, a neuro-transmitter that regulates physical exertion, mood swings and the attention span. By releasing endorphins, which inhibit pain and generate a 'feel-good' factor, this neuro-transmitter is instrumental in producing the feeling of euphoria experienced by athletes who are 'in the zone'.

The beneficial effects of endorphin release can be experienced by following my abdominal breathing method once an hour (see pages 36–48). Similar effects can be achieved by running at your own pace for 30 minutes each day (assuming you enjoy doing so), or by walking briskly for an hour, or by swimming for 30 minutes.

When you first start exercising, it may feel as if you have a mountain to climb and it is perhaps best to share the experience with a friend. Once you have exercised for several days, however, the endorphins will kick in; you will start to feel better and you will look forward to your daily exercise routine. What counts is taking that all-important first step.

Self-Massage

You can take the battle against depression into your own hands by the simple expedient of gently massaging your abdomen and head (see pages 123–7). Massage will help to establish two-brain harmony and, as a result, you will feel better and more relaxed, having promoted a sense of inner peace.

Abdominal Meditation

By directing your thoughts towards your abdomen you will break free from the vicious circle of negativity. Follow the recommended abdominal meditation routine (see page 128) for approximately ten minutes four or five times a day. After several weeks you should find that your depression lifts.

Diabetes, Type 2

I believe that poor abdominal health and nourishment are behind the spectacular growth in the number of people with diabetes. Diabetes has now reached epidemic proportions in Europe, with the number of people with diabetes approximately doubling over the past decade. Worse, there are many men, women and children who have diabetes without realising it. They might exhibit few if any of the classic symptoms (such as excess weight, slight fatigue or a compulsion to urinate frequently).

Diabetes may only be diagnosed by a doctor when serious and irreversible symptoms start to appear. These can include kidney problems, failing eyesight, inflammation of the artery walls, which can hinder circulation in the legs and lead to further complications, and the onset of cardiovascular disease.

If you have any family members with diabetes, you would be well advised to undergo tests to ascertain your blood sugar, blood pressure and cholesterol levels. These tests may reveal whether you have diabetes, or are likely to develop the condition, before complications appear.

Type 2 diabetes is present when there is a blood sugar count in excess of 1.26 g/litre. Sufferers' insulin receptors have become desensitised and the pancreas is forced to work overtime to generate additional insulin to metabolise blood sugar. Waist measurements in excess of 90 cm (35 in) for women and 100 cm (39 in) for men are key indicators of a heightened risk of diabetes. Losing weight will result in a reduction of abdominal fatty tissue and will improve insulin sensitivity and blood sugar levels. Some studies indicate that looking after the abdomen and reducing the amount of abdominal fatty tissue can cure up to 90 per cent of all cases of type 2 diabetes. If, after following my seven-step method for a period of three months, blood sugar levels have not returned to normal, further medical help should be sought.

Abdominal Breathing and Meditation

My abdominal breathing recommendations should be followed every hour (see pages 36–48) and abdominal meditation should be practised twice a day (see pages 128–33).

Exercises for the Two Brains

In order to shed excess fatty tissue around the waist, you are advised to follow my two-brain exercises as set out on pages 108–19. These have the additional benefit of strengthening the bile, liver and pancreatic tracts. The recommended two-brain exercise routine should be followed twice daily between meals.

Eating

My advice is as follows:

- Losing weight is the first priority but avoid low-calorie diets, which can cause fatigue and hyperglycaemia (an abnormally high concentration of sugar in the blood).
- Eat at regular intervals (light breakfast, lunch, mid-afternoon snack and dinner) to keep your blood sugar regulated. Eating indiscriminately and at irregular intervals will destabilise the metabolism and cause fatigue.
- Avoid snacking. According to a Canadian study published in the *British Medical Journal*, digestive disorders among adolescents with diabetes are two and a half times greater than those adolescents without diabetes. Females are particularly vulnerable, since they are more prone to fad dieting, bulimia and anorexia.
- Stop eating rich foods that cause weight gain. These include foods with a high sugar content (pastries, cakes, biscuits, white bread, pizzas, chocolate, honey, jams, sugary drinks and flavoured fizzy mineral water); foods with a high saturated fat content (hamburgers, hot-dogs, cold meats, bacon, fried butter, fermented or melted cheeses); and fibre supplements (pills and lozenges), together with foods with fibre additives (cereals, biscuits, bran) which, over time, irritate the intestinal lining.

- Never eat honey, jam or fruit on an empty stomach or drink fruit juices, tea or coffee, all of which can provoke hyperglycaemia.
- Alcohol stimulates the appetite and increases the calorie intake. The hyperglycaemic effects of alcohol depend on its sugar content. Avoid sweet drinks such as liqueurs and keep all alcohol consumption to a minimum. Drinking three or four glasses of wine is sufficient to provoke hyperglycaemia but two glasses of wine a day drunk with meals can be beneficial. Never drink alcohol on an empty stomach.
- Smoking, even moderately, heightens the body's need for insulin. There is only one option: stop smoking.
- Vary your food intake and eat healthy, high-quality foods, organic if you can afford it.
- Current research indicates that in most cases, carbohydrates should represent 50 per cent of the calorie intake. Where a person with diabetes is extremely overweight, the carb percentage should be reduced to around 40. Eat predominantly starchy foods such as wholemeal bread and cereals, pasta and rice. Eat fruit only in moderate quantities to avoid excessive fructose (fruit sugar) intake. Reduce the quantity of dairy products. During or at the end of a meal, eat raw or cooked green vegetables with a high vitamin content and plenty of natural fibre.
- Opt for mono-unsaturated fats, such as olive, rapeseed and groundnut oils. These should make up 25 per cent of the total calorie intake.
- Always eat slowly and in quiet surroundings. The pancreas, the organ which creates and regulates insulin, is hypersensitive to noise, stress and emotional factors.

Recreational Exercise

A sport practised for at least 30 minutes daily is more effective in reducing high blood sugar levels than the typical medication prescribed for type 2 diabetes.

- Opt for an endurance sport that appeals to you (see page 101) and practise it two or three times a week at your own pace. Why not try golf, cross-country skiing or roller blading? Walking at a sustained pace for 30 to 60 minutes a day is also beneficial.
- Take your children along and set an energetic example. Good habits are best learned early in life and, if you spend hours as a couch potato, sitting before a TV or computer screen, your

A sport practised for at least 30 minutes daily is more effective in reducing high blood sugar levels than the typical medication prescribed for type 2 diabetes.

children will follow your lead. Equally, if you take the lift, your kids are scarcely likely to walk upstairs instead. By the same token, if you get into your car to travel 500 metres (about 550 yards), your children will get out of the habit of walking.

Self-Massage

Manipulating the abdomen is extremely valuable for regulating insulin levels and eliminating cellulite. When the pancreas is not working optimally, there will be pain around the pancreatic plexus. The plexus and small intestine should be massaged (palpated, kneaded, pinched and rolled) for two to three minutes between meals (see pages 124 and 125).

People with diabetes often have poor oral hygiene, and are prone to gum disease. Professional dental care and finger-massaging the gums each morning can alleviate problems.

Fatigue

'Fatigue' is the term used to describe the state of permanent exhaustion that is rapidly emerging as the scourge of the age.[36] The condition tends to affect women more than men, perhaps because the former are called upon to assume a greater variety of responsibilities (domestic chores, child-rearing and professional life) and, in consequence, are exposed to a broader mix of hormonal and endocrinal fluctuations. There is statistical evidence to indicate that youngsters and those in active employment suffer more frequently from fatigue than those who have retired.

There can be a psychological factor in cases of fatigue: symptoms can be induced by professional cares, stresses and tensions. When fatigue manifests itself early in the week, it creates bad moods, decreased motivation, emotional swings, and general dissatisfaction. Morale is low and depression is imminent. Weekend fatigue tends to be more physical and typical consequences are forgetfulness, reduced attention span, lapses in concentration and various aches and pains such as abdominal cramps, aching joints and back pain. The week's workload has proved so stressful that the body clock is disrupted. Physical and intellectual effort has taken its toll. Eating patterns are irregular and recovery times insufficient.

Warning bells should start to ring if you feel unduly tired on holiday. This is frequently an indication of a chronic or infectious condition. Note that fatigue can also occur as a result of diabetes (see page 171), when blood sugar levels are extremely high.

High cholesterol levels can also cause fatigue and, left untreated, cardiovascular problems may result. In each instance, fatigue is essentially a shot across the bows – an unequivocal signal that your two brains are out of synch.

Eating

A fatigue-free day starts first thing in the morning. Follow my low-fat light breakfast routine (see page 94) for a period of three weeks, then switch to the energising breakfast (see page 96). Remember to eat slowly and while sitting down.

On no account should you start the day in haste or on an empty stomach, since this will disrupt your body clock and cause your digestive system to malfunction. Your appetite would then be unbalanced for the rest of the day, leading to snacking and/or skipped meals, which would give rise to bouts of fatigue and a lack of physical and mental well-being.

Take a three- to five-minute break every hour, using the time to practise abdominal breathing (see pages 36–48) or to drink a glass of water. The central nervous system 'runs down' every 50 minutes, resulting in lapses of concentration. It is important to take a short break at this point. If your physical or mental activity is too intense, eat a small snack between main meals, such as fruit, yoghurt, a slice of bread or a square of dark chocolate.

In the event of a sudden lapse in concentration, avoid biscuits, croissants, honey, jam or crisps, and avoid stimulants such as coffee, tea, alcohol or sugary drinks. Consuming sugar invariably leads to disruption of the metabolism, increases physical and mental fatigue and in the long-term can make you prone to type 2 diabetes.

PART III: TREATING COMMON CONDITIONS

As a general rule of thumb, eat healthy foods that appeal to you. Steamed or oven-baked dishes are best, typically served with a large quantity of aromatic herbs, fresh vegetables (raw or cooked), and seasonal fruits, which aid the digestion and contain lots of essential vitamins and minerals.

If you don't have a lot of time to eat, limit yourself to a main dish, ensuring that it always contains a serving of protein, carbohydrates and raw or cooked vegetables; alternatively, eat a wholemeal bread sandwich with a high protein and fresh salad content. When you come home from work, resist the temptation to indulge in a 'pick-me-up' (either alcohol or sugar-based drinks) and opt instead for a large glass of water.

Avoid cooking with butter, fried foods, sauces, cold meats, white flour products, hamburgers, pastries – in short, any foods that are likely to disrupt the digestive process and cause an imbalance between the first and second brains.

Recreational Exercise and Exercises for the Two Brains

Over the course of the day, try to walk or climb stairs at your own pace as often as you can. This will generate a rapid sense of well-being.

Choose your leisure-time activities with care, whether it's gardening, sport or DIY, and take a break every 20 minutes. It is essential not to exert additional pressure on yourself when you are already stressed: the result will only be to intensify fatigue and exacerbate pre-existing conditions (muscle cramps, painful joints, back pain, stomach upsets, and so on).

Take care not to fall into the trap of doing too much at the weekend, to the point that you go back to work on Monday thoroughly tired and worn-out. Over-exercising can result in symptoms of fatigue persisting over a period of weeks and may prove harmful to the body as a whole by making it vulnerable to viral infections.

To keep in shape, choose a recreational sport and practise it at least twice weekly at your own pace. If you opt for swimming, rest at first after each period of ten minutes; if walking or running, pause every 20 minutes; if cycling, every 30 minutes. You will find that this rhythm-based approach is more pleasurable and prevents morning-after exhaustion. Be careful to keep warm after exercise and take as much liquid refreshment as you feel necessary.

When you come home from work, resist the temptation to indulge in a 'pick-me-up' (either alcohol or sugar-based drinks) and opt instead for a large glass of water.

Abdominal Breathing and Self-Massage

When you come home from work, shower or take a bath, adding two handfuls of sea-salt to the water. Follow abdominal breathing exercises (see pages 36–48) and practise abdominal self-massage (pages 120–7). Salted hot-water massage is one of the best methods of combating fatigue and helping the body to relax both physically and mentally by ensuring two-brain harmony.

Massage can also focus on the head and feet; alternatively, indulge in a gentle full-body massage, with a qualified therapist or a willing partner.

Abdominal Meditation

Practise abdominal meditation twice daily (see pages 128–33). Remember that the abdomen is the source of energy and is directly linked to the upper brain. As such, its health dictates your overall mental and physical condition and well-being.

Flatulence

This condition, commonly referred to as 'wind', is caused by an excessive build-up of stomach gases. It is characterised by a distended stomach, cramps, a feeling of sluggishness, hyper-secretion

> **The condition is frequently a side effect of disorders such as nervous anxiety and always manifests itself after you have been eating or drinking too fast.**

of gastric juices, bad breath, general lassitude and, sometimes, chest pains which can be mistaken for symptoms of cardiac malfunction. The condition is frequently a side effect of disorders such as nervous anxiety and always manifests itself after you have been eating or drinking too fast. The symptoms should rapidly diminish and ultimately disappear if due attention is paid to abdominal health and the two-brain harmonisation approach is followed.

Abdominal Breathing

Repeating my breathe-to-relax sequence (see pages 46–8) five times before each meal will help you to relax and eat slowly. If you are eating in a restaurant, the routine can be practised while sitting and studying the menu. Avoid tight clothing and belts that constrict the abdomen.

Eating
- Don't eat quickly, in a noisy environment or while standing up.
- Limit your liquid intake: do not drink too much at one go, particularly in the case of fizzy or iced drinks.
- Never eat hunched over a low table.
- Never eat immediately after strenuous exercise or if you are perspiring heavily.
- Avoid eating so much that the stomach is distended.
- Avoid talking too much while eating.
- Note that chewing gum is a major cause of wind.
- Be careful to eat balanced meals and only eat in moderation the foods which are most likely to provoke wind: beans, lentils, fermented cheeses, melon, red fruits, tomatoes at the beginning of a meal, soups, pastries, honey and jam, mixed salad, sugary drinks. All of these ferment in the abdomen, causing bloating and flatulence.
- Moderate or eliminate entirely your intake of stimulants (tea, coffee, alcohol, tobacco), particularly when you are trying to lose weight.
- Break your daily food intake down into five light meals eaten in quiet surroundings and properly chewed.

Recreational Exercise
To prevent flatulence, it is important to relax the upper brain. One of the most efficient ways to do this is by practising your

choice of endurance sport for a maximum of 45 minutes at least two or three times a week (see page 101).

Self-Massage

Before sitting down to eat, practise a combination of my breathing exercises and follow a self-massage/*effleurage* routine (see pages 123–7). There is an 'aerophagic' point situated in the upper abdomen just below the ribs at the base of the solar plexus. This point should be massaged lightly, and can be done through your clothes if necessary.

Food Allergies

Food allergies are becoming increasingly prevalent.[37] You only have to look around you or consult the statistics. These allergies aggravate digestive disorders and cause problems such as vomiting, eczema and water retention. The incidence of food allergies has increased five times over the last two decades, particularly in young children. Respiratory allergies are also becoming more common (see the section on asthma on page 145).

When a patient complains of an allergic response, I habitually turn to his or her abdomen. The allergy may be food-related (the examples are legion) or respiratory (triggered by air pollution, pollen, dust mites, and causing asthma, sinusitis, eczema, pimples and pustules or stomach ailments). In almost every instance, an allergy will respond to treatment, will diminish over time and will frequently disappear if the abdomen is cared for and nurtured in accordance with the seven steps of my method.

Those who exhibit allergies tend to resort to medication, including the inevitable antihistamines. These generally result in an improvement in the patient's condition – but at what price? Anti-allergy medication always generates gastric hyperacidity which, in turn, provokes chronic indigestion and general fatigue in the upper brain. In fact, allergies always result from a poorly conditioned abdomen where the intestinal flora has been damaged. INSERM research at the Necker Clinic in Paris has recently demonstrated the link between intestinal disorders and the mechanics of allergic intolerance.

It is obvious that the first priority is to suppress the cause of the allergy in question. This will not suffice in the great majority of cases, however, because it is also necessary to reconstitute healthy intestinal flora and relax the upper brain. Only then will the allergy-related problems be relieved.

Eating

Dairy products, primarily cows' milk, are the root cause of numerous allergies. From the age of 45 onwards, three out of four people can no longer digest milk protein. Other allergens include eggs, peanut products, nuts in general, milk chocolate, shellfish and an ingredient called lupin flour that is sometimes used in biscuits. Other food allergies can be brought on by preservatives and additives such as inulin (a fructan or polysaccharide comprising fruit residues), an ingredient added for its fibre content and often found in butter, ice creams, yoghurt, cereals, jams and so on.

Certain other factors can make you more prone to food allergies: hyperacidity in the gut triggered by eating too fast and on an irregular basis; excessive intake of stimulants such as tea, coffee, alcohol or tobacco (even in the form of passive smoking); sustained ingestion of medication; or, quite simply, an excess of

PART III: TREATING COMMON CONDITIONS

pastries or cakes, notably those made using white flour. Other experts point to the dangers implicit in poor dental health.

It must be stressed that an allergenic product may cause harm when taken in normal quantities but can be tolerated by the system if ingested in smaller doses. In such cases, it may even work homeopathically to make you resistant to the allergen. My advice for combating allergies includes the simple expedient of varying the restaurants and shops you frequent as often as possible and consuming the freshest and most 'natural' foods available. Once again: eat in quiet surroundings, slowly and at regular intervals.

Abdominal Breathing

Abdominal breathing plays an important role in countering allergies as it enhances the circulation of the blood, thereby reducing excessive fermentation in the gut. Abdominal breathing can be practised at any time during waking hours (see pages 36–48).

Recreational Exercise

Used in conjunction with my breathe-to-relax method, recreational exercise reinforces the cardiovascular system and stimulates oxygenation of the blood, thereby helping to eliminate toxins in the abdomen, liver, glands and other organs. It is imperative that those prone to allergies warm up for a period of between five and seven minutes and that they 'cool down' over a ten-minute recovery period. Those with allergies should wear neither too many nor too few items of clothing in order to maintain a stable body temperature. Avoid over-strenuous exercises, since these can intensify an allergic response.

Exercises for the Two Brains

Two-brain exercises reinforce blood circulation in the abdomen and stimulate the proper functioning of the liver and the intestines, where toxins can accumulate.

Abdominal Meditation

Practise this at least once every day if you have food allergies (see page 128–33).

Gastritis

Gastritis is an inflammation of the stomach lining (the mucous membrane). The most obvious symptoms are heartburn, stomach cramp, nausea and a general sense of discomfort. Side effects include belching and bad breath.

All these can be traced back to an excess of acid in the stomach. This, in turn, is a result of stress, nervous tension, a poor diet, irregular food intake or chronic indigestion. If ignored or left untreated, gastritis can provoke stomach ulcers or colitis (see page 161). At all events, gastritis places an undue strain on the two brains.

Abdominal Breathing

Before sitting down to eat, a minimum of five minutes devoted to my abdominal breathing method (see pages 36–48) will help reduce tension and nervous anxiety.

Eating

Gastritis can be rapidly alleviated provided that you eat a varied antacid diet and that you take care to eat in moderation, slowly, and at regular intervals:

- Start the day with an antacid breakfast (see page 92).
- Do not sit down to eat if you are nervous or upset in any way.
- Eat in calm surroundings with the television set switched off.
- Eat at a table, taking care not to sit on too low a chair or to hunch over your food.
- Eat slowly to encourage the formation of saliva; chew your food properly.
- Avoid eating or drinking excessive quantities.
- Avoid fried or excessively spicy foods, acidic condiments such as vinegar, fruit juices (particularly on an empty stomach), fizzy water or drinks that are too hot or too cold.
- Avoid stimulants such as tea, coffee, tobacco and alcoholic spirits, particularly on an empty stomach.
- Avoid sugar-based foods (honey, jam, pastries, biscuits), all of which provoke excessive stomach acidity and induce gastritis.

Note: an infected tooth or inflammation of the gums may also result in excessive acidity. See your dentist.

Self-Massage

- First thing in the morning, brush your teeth and massage your gums with your fingers.
- Brush your teeth after each meal.
- Massage the solar plexus area regularly for two or three minutes at a time in order to eliminate cellulite build-up in the thorax and abdomen (see pages 124–5).

Self-massage helps you relax and relaxation is an essential weapon in the battle against gastritis.

Exercises for the Two Brains

Practise two-brain exercises (see pages 108–19) twice daily, once in the morning before breakfast and once again in the evening before dinner. Continue until the symptoms disappear, then follow the prescribed two-brain exercise routine each morning.

Abdominal Meditation

This is essential in all cases of gastritis, since excessive acidity can be alleviated by balancing the lower and upper brains. Surprisingly, the best time to practise abdominal meditation is before eating breakfast, when you are more often than not tense and in a hurry. (See page 132 for instructions.)

Headaches and Migraines

In many instances, headaches and migraines can be traced to an unhealthy abdomen, as they can be side effects of chronic indigestion, deficient intestinal flora, liver problems and/or an imbalance between the two brains. Migraines are caused by dilation and inflammation of the cranial arteries but it has not yet been decisively proved what causes this to happen.

Personally, I am convinced that the abdomen – the second brain – plays its part in these recurrent crises, since many migraine sufferers experience nausea and are prone to vomiting. I believe that the majority of headaches and migraines are caused by dysfunction at the level of the liver, bile and pancreatic tracts. By restoring abdominal health, I have frequently managed to reduce the frequency and intensity of headaches and migraines that have persisted for years. My breathe-to-relax routines, coupled with proper eating habits, recreational exercise and abdominal

PART III: TREATING COMMON CONDITIONS

breathing recommendations have proved effective in establishing the requisite harmony between the upper and lower brains. Migraine sufferers among my patients have responded in spectacular fashion and, in many instances, non-migraine headaches have disappeared for good.

Abdominal Breathing

Abdominal breathing routines are especially useful, since migraines and headaches occur more often among patients who are of a generally nervous disposition and prone to anxiety and high blood pressure. The abdominal breathing regime I recommend

> **I believe that the majority of headaches...are caused by dysfunction at the level of the liver, bile and pancreatic tracts.**

(see pages 36–48) effectively relaxes the upper brain by promoting the release of hormones that stimulate a sense of well-being. In numerous cases, this has resulted in a dramatic reduction in the incidence of headaches and migraines by preventing inflammation of the cranial arteries.

My abdominal breathing routine should be followed seven or eight times daily.

Eating

- Eat slowly, at regular intervals and in calm surroundings. Never skip meals (diets which prescribe a reduction in the number of meals will increase the incidence of headaches). Eating too much or ingesting stimulants such as alcohol or tobacco promote dilation of the blood vessels and can trigger a crisis.

- If you feel a headache or migraine coming on, immediately – but slowly – drink a cup of hot coffee or a glass of cold cola. However, don't do this after 3 or 4 pm.
- Avoid eating fatty or fried foods or those accompanied by sauces, together with cold meats, melted cheese, pastries or white flour products. Opt instead for vegetables, slow-acting sugars, fruit and fresh and natural produce.

Abdominal Meditation

Abdominal meditation regulates the arterial blood flow and relieves pain (see pages 128–33). In effect, the second brain – the abdomen – comes to the aid of the upper brain, where the headache appears to be located.

Insomnia

Sleep has its origins in both the upper brain and in the lower brain – the abdomen. The quality and duration of sleep are a function of two-brain harmony. Sleep patterns are conditioned by biorhythms developed since childhood, and our body clock is regulated to a large degree by the abdomen, which registers the various emotions, traumas and frustrations experienced in our early years. Our food intake therefore plays a key role in the quality of our nocturnal sleeping patterns.

Healthy sleep is essential to our overall balance, health and wellbeing. Sleeping in a darkened room encourages the secretion of melatonin, the hormone that alleviates the negative effects of insufficient sleep or 'jet-lag'. During sleep, the abdomen also plays its part in the secretion of serotonin, a neuro-transmitter stimulant, but an unhealthy abdomen produces either too much or too little serotonin – and the consequences can prove disastrous.

Recent research into the circadian cycle of alternating daytime activity and night-time rest has highlighted the role played by different areas of the upper brain in the cycles of REM (rapid eye movement) and non-REM sleep.[38] As yet, however, the activity of the lower brain – the abdomen – has not been thoroughly explored in this respect. That said, it is clear to me that abdominal activity during sleep must be in direct and complex correlation with the upper brain.

It has only recently been established that lack of sleep increases the risk of type 2 diabetes and can cause unwanted weight gain by disrupting the body's glucose and insulin levels. It has emerged that insomniacs secrete excess insulin and that those who 'sleep badly' are three times more likely to suffer from cardiovascular dysfunction.

To my mind, healthy sleep is impossible in the absence of a healthy abdomen. Accordingly, I have developed a series of recommendations to help combat insomnia by paying due attention to abdominal health.

Abdominal Breathing

Since we sleep for between a quarter and a third of our lives, by the age of 60 we will have spent roughly 20 years asleep. So healthy sleep must be a priority.

I recommend that you follow my breathe-to-relax exercises (see pages 46–8) before going to bed in a darkened room. On waking, it is important not to get out of bed too quickly. Instead, lie on your back, bend your legs and repeat my abdominal breathing routine five times. Use this time to plan the day ahead, and work out how you can build in some relaxation time. This is a key element in 'setting' your body clock.

Exercises for the Two Brains

Healthy and regenerative sleep patterns at night are a function of two-brain equilibrium during the day. Avoid any physical exercise that is too intense or that involves excessive muscular strain. In other words, no fast-paced games of squash, tennis, badminton or anything that is too competitive. Instead, relax your

...lack of sleep increases the risk of type 2 diabetes and can cause unwanted weight gain by disrupting the body's glucose and insulin levels.

two brains by practising yoga, light stretching exercises and abdominal meditation (see pages 128–33).

Eating

Good digestion is a prerequisite of good sleep. More often than not, disrupted sleep can be attributed to digestive conditions such as gastritis, flatulence, colitis and constipation. In such cases, it is essential to address the digestive condition first and foremost so consult the relevant section.

To ensure the proper functioning of the abdomen, it is important to eat slowly, at regular intervals, sitting down and in calm surroundings. Until your sleep improves, avoid any stimulants in the evening, such as tea, coffee, cola, alcohol or tobacco, together with all fast-acting sugars (honey, jam, biscuits, fruit juice). Eat a light dinner. Watch television selectively, avoiding programmes containing violence, and try to avoid switching channels over-frequently (this tires the eyes and, in consequence, the two brains).

Don't consume anything that could slow the digestive process and accelerate yeast build-up, such as soups (which dilate the stomach), excessive quantities of fruit and vegetables, fried foods, melted butter, cheeses (especially those with a high fat content) and stewed fruit. Do not drink to excess: one or two glasses of good wine over dinner can promote beneficial sleep, whereas three glasses can have the opposite effect.

Some foods are demonstrably conducive to a healthy sleep: apples, peaches, mangoes, bananas, yoghurt, a glass of milk, two squares of dark chocolate, chocolate mousse, or lightly steamed dishes. If you drink a herbal infusion, limit your intake to one cup; drinking more than one may result in your having to rise during the night to urinate. Avoid sleeping pills; these act on the upper brain and 're-set' the body clock, disrupting the absorption–elimination process at the level of the second brain. On no account should sleeping pills be taken on a regular basis: save them for exceptional circumstances (before an examination or post-trauma), because they will cause problems with your digestive transit and bowel movements.

Recreational Exercise

The choice of recreational exercise is an important factor. Gentle activities such as swimming or walking help alleviate abdominal problems caused by daytime stress. Extreme sports should be avoided; instead, exercise in moderation in calm, stress-free and pleasant surroundings. A 30-minute walk after dinner should help the digestive process and ensure a sound night's sleep.

Self-Massage and Abdominal Meditation

To achieve two-brain equilibrium – a precondition of sleeping well – I recommend a short period of face and head self-massage (see page 60) before going to bed, complemented by a three-minute routine of chest and abdomen massage. I have successfully treated a number of insomniac patients in this way.

Before you drop off to sleep I strongly recommend that you follow my abdominal meditation technique (see pages 128–33). Adhering to relaxation and self-massage routines has proved particularly efficacious in the case of lone yachtsmen who need to fine-tune their body clock and snatch a few hours of reinvigorating sleep irrespective of adverse weather and ocean conditions.

Sexual Problems

The upper and lower brains never interact more closely than during sexual intercourse. Desire is experienced in the upper brain and simultaneously in the abdominal region and if the two brains are not in synch, no release is possible. This accounts for sexual hang-ups, complexes, reduced arousal and other problems. Achieving sexual gratification is well-nigh impossible in the male and extremely difficult in the female in the absence of two-brain harmony. Making love successfully – or simply making love, period – is a pipe dream if the abdomen is in a poor condition. Diminished self-confidence leading to sexual failure and depression are typical consequences.

PART III: TREATING COMMON CONDITIONS

Conversely, a healthy abdomen interacting with the upper brain is receptive and conducive to sexual pleasure. Many sex-related problems in both men and women – such as diminished libido, difficulties in achieving and sustaining an erection, vaginal dryness, impotence, frigidity, premature ejaculation or pain during intercourse – can be solved by ensuring a properly functioning abdomen and reinstating two-brain harmony. This approach seems, to me at least, infinitely preferable and decidedly more 'natural' and effective than recourse to mega-vitamin treatments, aphrodisiacs, Viagra or any other medical stimulants which – despite all protestations to the contrary – have undesirable

Desire is experienced in the upper brain and simultaneously in the abdominal region and if the two brains are not in synch, no release is possible.

side effects. My conviction in this respect is reinforced by the recent conclusions reached by the redoubtable Professor Gershon, who has researched common sexual complaints (impotence, frigidity, sterility, etc.) and documented the role of molecular neurotransmitters common to both brains.

Abdominal Breathing

Abdominal breathing (see pages 36–48) generates relaxation and self-confidence, which are both key elements in the sex act, by freeing up and channelling abdominal energy and developing abdominal blood vessels. As a result, erection is more readily accomplished and vaginal lubrication intensified.

Exercises for the Two Brains

Practising abdominal movements has the effect of improving the circulation of blood in the entire digestive system. Blood flow to the lower abdomen is intensified, genital blood vessels are stimulated and there is heightened sensitivity in the perineal muscle (located between the anus and the scrotum or vulva). These effects can be stimulated by practising 10 to 20 pelvic floor contractions lasting up to 5 seconds and repeating them two or three times a day. The greater pelvic muscle strength will help give you more control over sexual response.

Self-Massage

Self-massage (see pages 120–7) is recommended to boost the libido and enhance your capacity to achieve orgasm. Massaging the skin soothes both body and mind; in some cases, impotence and frigidity can be relieved by very gentle massage before intercourse.

Eating

The upper brain blocks sexual gratification, and a poorly nourished abdomen can also prove a major impediment. Meals that are too big, too rich, too fatty or too 'liquid' in content will tire the two brains and, like alcoholic beverages and cigarettes, will inhibit sexual gratification. To make love well, it is important to eat selectively and in moderation (see page 70).

Abdominal Meditation

Many sexual problems can be traced back to traumatic events in the personal history of the individual concerned – and the abdomen will often carry the scars. Abdominal meditation is recommended to overcome these painful memories and engender a positive outlook. It also helps overcome the vicissitudes of everyday life which can affect and even totally inhibit sexual response – such as emotional stress, anxiety, social pressures, self-doubt, shyness, loneliness, poor communication skills. By reconciling the two brains and re-establishing emotional stability, abdominal meditation will help you to feel closer to your partner, foster openness and pave the way for a life of sexual intimacy that is securely anchored in two-brain health (see pages 128–33).

Unwanted Weight Gain

More than 20 per cent of British adults are obese, and the number of obese children is rising faster here than in the United States. The major factors that have resulted in the extra weight piling on can all be traced to the abdomen. It is here that stress, emotional problems, anxieties and frustrations are manifest, causing digestive disorders such as bulimia, compulsive snacking, cravings, and addiction to foods that are too rich, fatty and/or sugary. The body fails to eliminate these substances and they accumulate, causing the abdomen to become distended and prone to cramps.

Restoring two-brain harmony and regularising the absorption–elimination process will inevitably lead to sustainable weight loss. The abdomen is more than a simple food-processing plant; it is also the source of immune cells and neuro-transmitters that perform complex functions linked to and harmonised with the upper brain. Thus, by treating the abdomen, you can also improve mental conditions such as anxiety, shyness and hypersensitivity – all of which contribute to unwanted weight gain.

Eating

While you are slimming, always eat slowly and selectively, at regular intervals.

- Take a hot shower every morning, then use a towel to dry your waist and abdomen vigorously in order to stimulate the liver, pancreas and bile ducts. Brush your teeth, massage the gums with your fingers to remove any impurities lodged there during the night and stimulate the production of saliva, then you will be ready for the first meal of the day.
- Eat breakfast roughly 15 minutes after waking up. Do *not* breakfast in bed: eating when lying down obstructs the digestive tracts and leads to a build-up of fats. By the same token, skipping breakfast results in an over-secretion of bile and a surfeit of insulin which, with nothing on hand to process, causes excessive stomach acid.
- Eat at regular intervals and only at proper meal times; stick to three meals per day – or three meals plus one or two small snacks depending on the amount of energy you use during the working day.
- Dinner should be the *lightest* meal of the day in order to avoid accumulation of fats and to prevent digestive problems. At dinner, avoid soups, an excess of raw vegetables, cheeses and sugar-based desserts.
- Scientific research has established that we tend to require the same quantity of nutrients at each meal in order to assuage our hunger. If you are reducing your overall calorie intake, you

need to choose foods with great care and to opt for those that are less rich, less fatty and less sugary than what you ate previously. Thus, if two yoghurts are on offer – one plain, one with fruit – *always* choose the former so as to reduce the sugar content. Similarly, when two meat dishes are available, always opt for the lighter of the two, preferably grilled and without a sauce.

• Avoid all sugary drinks; each glass contains the equivalent of two to three lumps of sugar. Avoid alcoholic beverages generally and especially those with a high alcohol content. Limit yourself to at most one glass of wine or beer with each meal. Drink water – 2 litres ($3^1/_2$ pints)– throughout the day and especially to accompany meals.

• If you must drink coffee or tea, restrict your intake to a single cup – but never on an empty stomach or after 5 pm..

Abdominal Breathing

My abdominal breathing method (see pages 36–48) and the resultant 'natural' abdominal massage have many benefits for those who want to lose unwanted weight. The routine helps to regulate digestive functions and, by encouraging the release of endorphins, induces relaxation at the level of the upper brain. Follow my abdominal breathing routine before each meal (or snack) to aid the digestive process and before you go to sleep.

Recreational Exercise and Exercises for the Two Brains

It is impossible to lose weight and keep it off without indulging in some physical activity that is appropriate to your age, overall physical condition and preferences. Movements must be regulated by your breathing patterns, which are designed to reinforce the cardiovascular system, improve the circulation and to siphon off and eliminate excess fats via the abdomen and other organs. It is vital that the physical movements involved are regular and co-ordinated, and that they do not over-stress the heart, or the effect will be the reverse of that intended. The exercises outlined for the two brains (pages 108–19) are designed in such a way that they will induce relaxation in the upper brain as well as helping you to shed unwanted weight.

Endurance sport will boost the cardiovascular system and improve your muscle tone and physique. Medical research has established that the breakdown of fatty reserves begins after 45 minutes of exercise. The important thing is to ensure that fat is eliminated without detriment to muscle. Indulge in recreational exercise at least three times weekly. Be careful to stop at the first signs of fatigue or shortness of breath. In that case, postpone the exercise until the following day.

Self-Massage

Weight gain is accompanied by digestive dysfunction. Self-massage, particularly when directed at the appropriate plexus, enhances the circulation and stimulates glands and organs which, when functioning optimally, eliminate toxins and prevent the accumulation of unwanted fats. Abdominal self-massage also helps relax the upper brain. (See pages 120–7 for instructions).

Abdominal Meditation

Abdominal meditation contributes substantially to the elimination of unwanted weight (see pages 128–33). It helps reconcile the upper and lower brains and combats the negative effects of stress, nervous anxiety and emotional disorders, all of which prompt weight gain. Meditating in the early evening can aid the digestive process and foster a healthy sleep, which in itself is an important factor in the slimming process.

Looking Your Best

'Beauty' may well be in the eye of the beholder but in my opinion it is essentially abdomen-deep. A healthy abdomen is a precondition of beautiful skin and luxuriant hair, good teeth, a flat stomach, a cellulite-free body, firm hips and buttocks and a slender waist. A harmonious relationship between brain and abdomen is indispensable to a stable, balanced, serene and self-confident lifestyle. In other words, 'beauty' is contingent on both brains.

The link between abdominal health and external beauty is explained by the fact that the abdomen is the source of nourishment for the body. Skin cells require replenishment at a much faster rate than kidney or liver cells but, since they are effectively at the end of the distribution chain, they are the first to show signs of wear and tear.[39]

The vitamins that are a prerequisite of 'beauty' can be destroyed in the intestinal tract if the abdomen is unhealthy. Intestinal flora must not be subject to excessive fermentation (which gives rise to chronic indigestion) but, instead, they should be capable of absorbing and distributing vitamin intake throughout the body and eliminating toxins.

Time and again, I have treated women who, despite eating prudently, slowly and at regular intervals, nonetheless exhibit major skin problems. Typically, they attempt to address those problems by applying creams and lotions or resorting to medication. On examination, however, they have all exhibited an abdomen that is distended and painful – a sure-fire indication of chronic indigestion. Once their abdominal health is restored, their skin takes on a new glow, wrinkles and crow's feet disappear, and dry hair acquires a fresh sheen. Hair loss is a thing of the past and the various creams and lotions they apply to their skin can now do their job more effectively.

Treating the abdomen is the first major step on the road to boosting the immune system and curing skin disorders such as eczema, psoriasis and persistent acne.

A healthy abdomen is a precondition of beautiful skin and luxuriant hair, good teeth, a flat stomach, a cellulite-free body, firm hips and buttocks and a slender waist.

Eating

In order to nourish the external body cells – skin, hair and nails – and prevent skin from ageing, the abdomen must be capable of absorbing and processing essential antioxidants which target free radicals (see pages 87, 88 and 89) and certain essential oils. A straightforward first step is to cut back on sugar consumption, as it triggers excessive intestinal fermentation and leads to unsightly cellulite.

Group B vitamins are front-line troops in the battle for beauty:

B_1, also known as thiamin, is an antioxidant that ensures proper absorption of carbohydrates and the conversion of fat into energy.

B_2, in conjunction with Vitamin A, is essential for cellular health and a major factor in promoting healthy skin, nails and hair.

B_3, also known as niacin, ensures proper oxygenation and acts as a shield against harmful UV rays.

B_5 is an antioxidant that reduces ageing; this is the most important of the B group vitamins in this context, as it protects skin, nails and mucous membranes.

B_6 is an antioxidant that regulates skin secretions; deficiency can cause hair loss and eczema.

B_8 is essential for the circulation and for healthy skin; deficiency can cause hair loss and dermatitis.

B_9 helps boost red blood cell formation as part of the immune system; it promotes cell replication and skin renewal.

B_{12} helps improve skin tone, colour and luminosity.

B group vitamins are present in:
- wholegrain cereals, yeast, wheatgerm
- pulses and soya products
- fresh green vegetables, including spinach, courgettes, cabbage, lettuce, leeks and green beans, together with garlic, onions, mushrooms and avocado
- lean meat and offal: liver, kidneys, brains, sweetbreads
- poultry
- fish and shellfish: tuna, cod, sole, sardines, crab, shrimps, oysters
- eggs
- dairy produce: milk, cheese
- nuts
- bananas, dates, figs.

The principal aggressors that affect our looks are alcohol taken in immoderate quantities or other stimulants such as tobacco. Over-exposure to the sun can lead to skin cancer, the incidence of which is increasing.

Abdominal Breathing

Abdominal breathing is a beauty aid because it accelerates the elimination of toxins and retards skin ageing by helping the circulation of dedicated fibre-secreting cells in connective tissue, known as fibroblasts. These help collagen retention and, as a result, work against the formation of wrinkles. My breathe-to-relax recommendations (see pages 46–8) should be followed.

Exercises for the Two Brains

A flat and well-muscled abdomen is aesthetically pleasing. To maintain (or develop) a flat abdomen, nothing works better than my two-brain exercise routines (see pages 108–19). They will help to eliminate excessive abdominal fermentation, chronic indigestion and cellulite. A key element in this process is the visualisation of yourself with a slimmer figure and the satisfaction and self-confidence that such a figure will project.

Self-Massage

Self-massage of the face, head and abdomen is particularly recommended. Massaging the face and head (see page 60) works on the cranial and vagus nerves, soothes the central nervous system, imparts energy and instils a sense of relaxation which helps eliminate tension – and wrinkles. Self-massage tones and softens the skin, reduces 'bags' under the eyes (often a symptom

PART III: TREATING COMMON CONDITIONS

of liver disorders) and dissipates unwanted rolls of fat (often symptoms of digestive dysfunction).

Abdominal self-massage (see pages 120–7) helps develop the blood vessels in the skin and eliminate impurities as well as promoting abdominal flexibility and suppressing cellulite build-up. Abdominal self-massage is good for the body as a whole, and not just the particular area being targeted.

Recreational Exercise

Exercise affects the way we look by eliminating abdominal tension, enhancing deep and peripheral circulation, and stimulating the various systems that stop toxins lodging in the tissues. A healthy and attractive body is difficult to maintain without regular exercise in the form of an endurance sport (see page 101). Walking, cycling, swimming, cross-country skiing, golf, roller blading and other pastimes are all effective beauty aids.

Abdominal Meditation

Attractiveness in both sexes also comes from *inside,* as a reflection of your personality. The abdominal meditation routines I recommend (see pages 128–33) help to reveal your true inner self, substituting the real for the purely cosmetic, the underlying essence for the superficial appearance. The key is to become at one with yourself by ensuring harmony between the upper and lower brains.

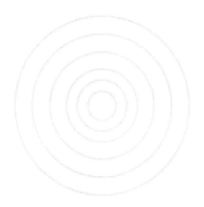

CONCLUSION

I was pleasantly surprised when I discovered that medical science had formally demonstrated what I have long known to be true and what I have practised in all my years as a therapist: that everything stems from the abdomen and, in the absence of harmony between the abdomen and the upper brain, no treatment can be successful.

When something goes wrong, people tend to consult doctor after doctor, experimenting with one regimen after another, from medication to spa treatments, whereas the real answer lies within. I trust my approach has demonstrated that you are your own best therapist. In modern society it's hard to find time for genuine one-to-one communication, and there's a tendency to become ensconced in front of the TV set or the computer, slaves to advertising and stereotyping. My method frees up time to eat, think, dream, love and take exercise as you see fit.

Each of the seven basic tenets of my method is the result of many years' reflection, but each is easy to put into practice. I have made allowance for social pressures, schedules, travel – in short, the constraints imposed by modern life – at the same time as showing how to address your complaints and disorders and prevent even more serious illness.

I am astonished at the results I see each day as I treat patients for such diverse ailments as back pain, fatigue, depression, cardio-vascular disorders, diabetes, unwanted weight gain or loss, insomnia and abdominal complaints such as constipation, colitis or period pain. And I am sorely tempted to ask why those in charge of a nation's health do not react more positively. At the moment it seems there is insufficient awareness of the best ways to address the functional disorders that poison our lives and how we can help medical practitioners treat and cure those disorders.

Do you want to live a healthy life or are you content to remain dependent on medication, fashionable wonder products and miracle cures? As far as miracles are concerned, the ball is firmly in your own court.

I hope this book is helpful in persuading you to take greater control over your own health. All it takes is to change a few ingrained habits and perhaps acknowledge that you can and must adjust. It may be that you were unaware of what you are doing wrong and how disastrous the consequences could be. I can only hope that my approach to sustained abdominal health and two-brain harmony will open your eyes to a new way of living and to a fresh awareness of health and well-being.

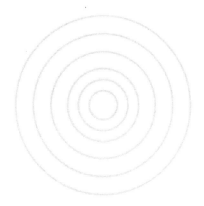

SOURCES

1. Michael D. Gershon, *The Second Brain: A Groundbreaking New Understanding of Nervous Disorders of the Stomach and Intestine*, Harper Paperbacks, 1999.

2. Dr Emmanuel de Viel, 'Des récepteurs au goût amer dans l'estomac et l'intestin', published in *Le Quotidien du Médecin*, N° 7069, pp. 2392–7, 19 February 2002.

3. Boris Dolto was a kinesiologist and teacher of manual therapies, as well as the founder of the Cujas school in Paris. He was married to the famous psychoanalyst Françoise Dolto, author of several works on children.
Boris J. Dolto, *Le corps entre les mains*, Editions Hermann, Paris, 1988. (Chapter X, 'l'Ame du ventre', pages 249–55)
Françoise Dolto, *Autoportrait d'une psychanalyste, 1934–1988*, Editions du Seuil, October 1989.

4. Joseph Kessel, *Les Mains du miracle*, Editions Gallimard, Paris.

5. Dr Emmanuel de Viel, 'L'alimentation aurait une influence directe sur la fonction respiratoire', *Le Quotidien du Médecin* N° 6749, 1 September 2000. Florence, World Congress of Respiratory Diseases.

6. Gérard Tortora (Bergen Community College) and Sandra Reynolds Grabowski (Purdue University), *Principles of Anatomy and Physiology*, 3rd French edition, translated from the 9th American edition, Editions DeBoeck Université. Page 502, 'Survey of the cranial nerves'.

7. Carol Krucoff, 'Breathe. You Think You Know How to Do It. You're Wrong', published in the *Washington Post*, 2 May 2000. At Duke University Medical Center, nurse Jon Seskevich has taught abdominal breathing to more than 15,000 patients.

8. Dr Isabelle Catala, 'Le taux de cholestérol s'élève moins si on fractionne les repas', *Le Quotidien du Médecin* N° 7022, 3 December 2001. Ref: *British Medical Journal*, vol. 323, pp. 1286–8, 1 December 2001.

9. Dr Denise Caro, 'Fractionnement des repas ne veut pas dire grignotage', *Le Quotidien du Médecin* N° 6968, 17 September 2001. Symposium organised by the centre for research LU under the auspices of the 17th International Congress of Nutrition in Vienna.

10. Dr Denise Caro, 'Adapter l'alimentation aux rythmes de travail', *Le Quotidien du Médecin* N° 6773, Cahier 2 Nutrition N°11, 5 October 2000, page 26.

11. 'L'axe hypothalamo-hypophysaire impliqué dans la boulimie nocturne', *Le Quotidien du Médecin* N° 7066, 14 February 2002. In nocturnal bulimia, 50 per cent of the food is absorbed after 20 hours. Ref: *American Journal of Physiology-Endocrinology and Metabolism*, 12 February 2002.

12. Dr Catherine Desmoulins, 'Ramadan: l'heure des repas pourrait modifier les sécrétions hormonales', *Le Quotidien du Médecin* N° 6905 25 April 2001.
Ref: André Bogdan, Belal Bouchareb, Yvan Touitou, *Life Sciences* 68 (2001): 1607–1615.

13. Dr Béatrice Vuaille, 'La nutrition est un important facteur de régulation hormonale', *Le Quotidien du Médecin* N°6799, 13 November 2000.
Paper by Dr Jacques Bringer (head of endocrine illnesses at the Lapeyronie Hospital, Montpellier) to the European congress 'Woman and Nutrition' organised by CERIN (Centre for Research and Nutritional Information).

14. Marie-Christiane Moreau INRA, Jouy-en-Josas, 'Microflore intestinale, prébiotiques, probiotiques et immunomodulation', 2001, volume 6, NAFAS Science.

Bulletin of the database NUTRIPID et CERINUT, 'Les probiotiques: des microorganismes bénéfiques pour notre système
immunitaire?', Numéro 63 of January/February 2001.

Institut Danone factsheet, 'L'intestin, cet inconnu', Nutrition N°
65, septembre 2002.

Entretiens de Bichat, 'L'intestin intelligent', report of 26 September
2002)

Dr Denise Caro, 'L'intestin, un bouclier contre les agressions', Le
Quotidien du Médecin N° 7228 , Cahier 2, 28 November 2002,
Nutrition N° 20.

10th International Congress of Bacteriology and Applied
Microbiology, sponsored by Danone Vitapole.

15. Dr Anne Teyssédou-Mairé, 'Diabète, une épidémie mondi-
ale', Le Quotidien du Médecin N° 7020, Cahier 2 Nutrition N°16,
29 November, pages 5, 6, 7, 8, 9.

Christian Delahaye, 'L'Institut de veille sanitaire publie les dernières
données épidémiologiques. Diabète de type 2: les généralistes
pour relever le défi', Le Quotidien du Médecin N° 7127, 17 Mai
2002.

American study following a group of 9,665 people aged 25 to 74
years, who were recorded from the age of 20: 'Des fruits et des
légumes pour diminuer l'incidence du diabète de type 2', Le
Quotidien du Médecin N° 6910, Cahier 2 Nutrition N°14, 3 May
2001, page 48. (E.S. Ford, Prev Med; 32 (1): 33–39).

16. 'Intolérance au lactose ou allergie aux protéines du lait', Le
Quotidien du Médecin-Nutrition, page 18, 19 October 2000.

17. Dr Guy Benzadon, 'Sucré, salé. Le sucre, ni faux ni vrai ennemi. Tout, tout on saura tout sur les glucide', *Le Quotidien du Médecin* N° 7424, 13 November 2003.
Ref: Dr Jacques Fricker (Bichat hospital, Paris) and Dr Philippe Passa (diabetes specialist, Saint-Louis hospital, Paris) for the AFSSA (Agence française de sécurité sanitaire des aliments).

18: Dr Béatrice Vuaille, 'Alcool et cerveau: mieux vaut boire peu que pas du tout', *Le Quotidien du Médecin* N° 6963, 10 September 2001.
Ref: American alcohol study (Keneth Mukamal et al., Boston).

19: Dr Annie Dumonceau, 'Le goût, entre inné et acquis', from 'Cet apprentissage du goût comporte bien sûr des aspects biologiques, psychologiques, sociaux et culturels', *Le Quotidien du Médecin* N° 6773, Cahier 2 Nutrition N°11, 5 October 2000, page 17.

20. Dr Mathilde Ferry, 'L'apprentissage du goût, une étape fondamentale chez l'enfant', *Le Quotidien du Médecin* N° 6689, 17 April 2000.
With Dr France Belliste, 'L'apprentissage du goût se fait dès la prime enfance', INSERM U341, Hôtel-Dieu, Paris.
Summary by Dr Daniel Rigaud, 'L'analyse de l'apprentissage du goût est primordiale pour comprendre les troubles du comportement alimentaire', Bichat hospital, Paris.
Today, anorexia, bulimia and compulsive eating are most often encountered in adolescents. They are the expression of an illness of which the symptoms are fear of eating too much, extreme

underweight or regular vomiting. Treatment of these problems must be nutritional, behavioural and psychotherapeutic.

21. Ludmila Couturier, 'L'idée d'une nutrition préventive fait son chemin', *Le Quotidien du Médecin*, 11 December 2001.
According to Professeur Serge Renaud (INSERM), following the Cretan diet has resulted in a significant reduction in deaths due to coronary heart disease. Ref: IFOP survey covering a representative group of 1,002 members of the French public and 200 members of the medical profession (120 GPs and 80 specialists).
Dr Denise Caro, 'Aliments: l'allégation santé, concept à utiliser avec précaution', *Le Quotidien du Médecin*, N° 7062, 8 February 2002.
Ref: The recognition of the effects on health of certain foods in a countrywide campaign to educate the public and doctors about the medical benefits of preventative nutrition, by the PNNS (Programme national nutrition santé).
Dr Michel de Lorgeril, La Tronche, '4ème rencontres de nutrition. Le régime méditerranéen: un modèle de prévention. L'association des effets cardioprotecteurs et des effets bénéfiques sur le bilan lipidique confère au régime méditerranéen un intérêt considérable dans la prévention des cardiopathies', *Le Quotidien du Médecin* N° 6784, 20 October 2000.

22. Report by Dr Béatrice Vuaille and Dr Isabelle Catala, 'Thé ou café ? Le thé paré de vertus à vérifier. Le catalogue des méfaits et bienfaits du café', *Le Quotidien du Médecin* N° 7675, 27 January 2005.

23. 'Le jour où la France se mit à fumer, elle commença à s'empoisonner', *Le Quotidien du Médecin, Histoire de la Médecine*, pages 18–20, 21 November 2002.

24. The SUVIMAX Study (supplementation with antioxidant vitamins and minerals) co-ordinated by Dr Serge Hercberg, Director of Research at INSERM (Institut Scientifique et Technique de la Nutrition et de l'Alimentation) has just finished. This French study, which lasted 8 years, covered 13,027 subjects – 7,886 women aged 35 to 60 and 5,141 men aged 45 to 60 – who had taken a daily supplement. One group received a placebo and the others a cocktail of antioxidants: betacarotene, vitamin C, vitamin E, selenium and zinc. Early results in 2001 showed that the French population as a whole were deficient in vitamins C, D and E, iron, iodine and magnesium. The final results demonstrated that taking antioxidants reduced the risk of getting cancer by 31 per cent and lessened the mortality rate among men. This result didn't apply to women until they increased their consumption of fruits and vegetables. One in three cancers could be avoided. In conclusion, the nutritional recommendations for cancer prevention of eating a minimum of five fruits and vegetables a day are confirmed. Dr Serge Hercberg's study only covered natural supplementation.

25. Dr Emmanuel de Viel, 'Vitamines: mise en garde américaine contre les supplémentations abusives', *Le Quotidien du Médecin* N° 6691, 19 April 2000.
British Medical Journal, 18 March 2000, p. 813.

26. Dr Béatrice Vuaille, 'La clé de l'effet antidépresseur de l'exercice physique', *Le Quotidien du Médecin*, 2001
British Journal of Medicine, 2001: 35: 342–343.

27. Dr Martine Perez, 'Diabète: Une étude américaine démontre les bienfaits de l'exercice physique dans la prévention du diabète gras chez les personnes à risque' ; 'Le sport plus efficace que le médicament';. 'Les médecins ont sélectionné 3,234 personnes non diabétiques mais à risque', articles in *Le Figaro, Sciences et Médecine*, 9–10 February 2002.
Ref: *New England Journal of Medicine*, 7 February 2002.
Dr Véronique Nguyen, 'Régime et exercice: c'est prouvé on peut prévenir le diabète de type 2', *Le Quotidien du Médecin* N° 6911, 4 May 2001. Report on the Finnish Diabetes Prevention Study covering 523 subjects of at least 55 years of age.
Ref: *New England Journal of Medicine*, 3 May 2001, pp. 1343 and 1390.
Dr Jean-Michel Borys, 'Prévention du diabète de type 2: le succès du régime et du sport', *Le Quotidien du Médecin* N° 6782, 18 October 2000.
Ref: Congress of the ADA, based on a report by the DPP Study Group Rock Ville, by Drs T. Gaillard (Colombus), Darra (Colombus), and Holman (Oxford).

28. Dr Véronique Nguyen (New York correspondent), *Sciencexpress*, 16 December 2004, published as 'Une découverte de taille dans la graisse viscérale, une hormone qui agit comme l'insuline', *Quotidien du Médecin*, December 2004.

A Japanese study led by Dr Iichiro Shimomura (University of Osaka), found that new adipose tissues is created preferentially by the surface layer of abdominal fat.
Ref: Pierre Pallardy, *Mon code de vie*, éditions Robert Laffont, 2005. Pages 33–4.

29. Recollections by Aniela Jaffé, *C.G. Jung, ma vie: souvenirs, rêves et pensées*, translated from German by Dr Roland Cahen, Collection Témoins, Editions NRF Gallimard, 1973. Originally published as *Erinnerungen, Träume, Gedanken*, Rascher, Zurich and Stuttgart, 1962.

30. Odile Jacob (ed.), *Les vilains petits canards*, 2001; *Le murmure des fantômes*, 2003; *Parler d'amour au bord du gouffre*, 2004.

31. Dr Dominique Brillaud, 'Le ventre siège des émotions', *Le Quotidien du Médecin*, N° 6772, 4 October 2000.
Ref: 'Les troubles banals du transit…Le ventre vit sous l'emprise de l'affectif…un peu d'ostéopathie peuvent aider les victimes de tous ces maux': report in the magazine *Alternative Santé/ L'Impatient*, September 2000.

32. 'Alimentation anticancer: la preuve par 500,000 sujets', *Le Quotidien du Médecin* N° 6943, 25 June 2001. It's not a new idea that nutrition can help to prevent cancer, but it was confirmed by the EPIC (European Prospective Investigation into Cancer and Nutrition) study released in 1991 by the CIRC de Lyon, which gathered data on 500,000 subjects in ten countries. The first results, present at the Nutrition and Cancer conference in

Lyons, showed evidence for the protective effects of fish, fruits and vegetables.

'Cancers: de nombreux travaux sur le rôle des facteurs nutritionnels', *Le Quotidien du Médecin* N° 6970, 19 September 2001. Eurocancer was a symposium dedicated to finding a metabolic and nutritional approach to cancer treament, co-organised by the scientific committee APRIFEL.

33. Dr Denise Caro. 'Prévention cardio-vasculaire: les cinq règles diététiques', *Le Quotidien du Médecin* N° 6899, 17 April 2001. Ref: Symposium organised by Fruit d'or research (Unilever).

34. Dr Véronique Nguyen (New York correspondent), 'L'exercice régulier combat l'athérosclérose en abaissant la protéine C réactive', *Le Quotidien du Médecin* N° 7010, 15 November 2001. Ref: Congress of the American Heart Association (Anaheim), 74th Session. Report by Dr Rainer Raurama (Kuopio Research Institute of Sports Medicine, Finland).

35. 'Alimentation et syndrome de l'intestin irritable', *Le Quotidien du Médecin* N° 6910, Cahier 2, Nutrition N° 14, page 49. Ref: M. Simren, *Digestion*, 63 (2): 108–115.

36. Dr Annie Dumonceau, 'La fatigue: un mal qui touche près de la moitié des français', *Le Quotidien du Médecin* N° 6774, 6 October 2000. Ref: a study by Laboratoires Therval/ IPSOS/ Le Quotidien Santé. Dr Janine Defrance, 'Les trois profils de patients fatigués', *Le Quotidien du Médecin* N° 7197, 14 October 2002.

Ref: Paris. Press conference held by the Laboratoires Whitehall France.

37. 'Devant la recrudescence des allergies alimentaires, la création d'un système d'allergovigilance', *Le Quotidien du Médecin* N° 6701, 5 May 2000.
Ref: *Journée Nationales de la Société Française d'Allergologie et d'Immunologie Clinique.* Following a report by Prof. D.A. Moneret-Vautrin (Nancy).

38. Dr Janine Defrance, 'Une journée internationale pour l'éducation sur le sommeil', *Le Quotidien du Médecin* N° 6869, 5 March 2001.
Ref: 1st International Sleep Conference, 21 March 2001, organised by the International Foundation for Mental Health and Neurosciences: 'Open your eyes to sleep'. Sleep problems affect 70 million Americans.
Dr Martine André, 'Comment aider les patients atteints de troubles du sommeil', *Le Quotidien du Médecin* N° 7106, 12 April 2002. Ref: 'Aider vos patients à retrouver le sommeil', France.

39. Dr Denise Caro, 'La peau se nourrit de vitamines et d'acides gras', *Le Quotidien du Médecin* N° 6696, Cahier 2, Nutrition N°10, 27 April 2000, pages 53–4.
Ref: Dr Patrick Serog, *La diététique et la peau* , Editions du Rocher. 'Actualités et Recherches en Nutrition Cutanée', special report by Dermatologie et Nutrition (Vichy).

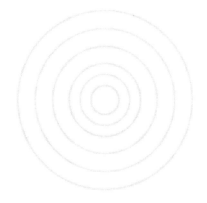

ABOUT THE AUTHOR

PIERRE PALLARDY is an osteopath, dietician and physical therapist and has been successfully treating patients with various physical and mental ailments for more than 30 years. He specialises in back pain, slimming, stress management and sleep problems. He and his wife are based on the Île de Ré off the west coast of France, where they run wellness holidays.

To find out more about Pierre Pallardy and his work, visit his website *www.domainedelabaronnie.com*. For more books by Pierre Pallardy (in French) see *www.pallardy.com*.

By the same author

La grande forme, Encre, 1979

En pleine santé, Édition° 1, 1981

Manger pour guérir, RMC Éditions, 1985

La forme naturelle, Édition° 1, 1986
Les chemins du bien-être, Fixot 1990
Le droit au plaisir, Fixot, 1992
Le cri du cœur, Plon, 1996
Maigrir là où vous voulez, Édition° 1, 1999
Maigrir sans regrossir, Édition° 1, 2000
Plus jamais mal au dos, Éditions Robert Laffont, 1988, 2001
Vaincre fatigue, stress, déprime et protéger son cœur, Éditions Robert Laffont, 2003
Mon code de vie: santé, jeunesse, harmonie, Éditions Robert Laffont, 2005

Author's acknowledgement
My deepest thanks go to my wife Florence, a constant source of support throughout the past 35 years, who has subordinated her own artistic endeavours to help me communicate my deeply held convictions. My efforts in that respect will have been rewarded if I succeed in persuading readers to take responsibility for their own health and well-being.

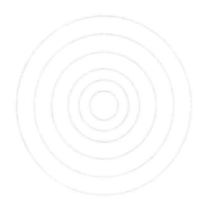

INDEX

Main page entries are highlighted in bold